Advance Praise for

ALZHEIMER'S DISEASE AND OTHER DEMENTIAS

The Caregiver's Complete Survival Guide

"**At last, a roadmap for those who care for someone with memory loss.** Nataly Rubinstein has given us an utterly human view of what it's like for a person and their family dealing with Alzheimer's disease. Going far beyond a clinical explanation, she provides insight into the deepest concerns we all share maintaining these individuals' lives and dignity and gives caregivers the confidence to know how to meet these needs."
 —Raul Grosz, MD
 Board-certified neurologist
 Neuroscience Consultants, Aventura and Miami Beach, Florida

"**An invaluable treasure of practical advice and compassionate understanding.** This indispensable book will guide you through the complexities, the responsibilities, and the challenges all caregivers face. Written by a remarkable woman, with wit and a human touch, it gives one encouragement and hope for one's own survival."
 —Sabina Shalom
 Caregiver for her husband, Mark
 Author of *A Marriage Sabbatical*

"An **extremely insightful, knowledgeable, but also easy-to-read and comforting** book. I would recommend it to anyone who has concerns about the possibility that their loved one is living with Alzheimer's or dementia."
—Gary Edward Barg
Author of *The Fearless Caregiver*
Founder and editor in chief of *Today's Caregiver* magazine

"**Nataly's advice has kept me from jumping off the edge!** She can always take the worst-case scenario and spin it into something positive and workable."
—Julia B. Sosnick
Full-time caregiver for her husband, Phil

"This book is **truly the caregiver's GPS** for navigating the long and arduous road of Alzheimer's. The educational benefit to the caregiver and family of anyone affected by this disease is unmatched by anything I have seen in my seventeen years of dealing with Alzheimer's. I look forward to recommending the book to everyone I meet who may in any way be touched by Alzheimer's."
—Larry E. Butcher
Former chair, Alzheimer's Disease Advisory Committee, State of Florida
Member, board of directors, Alzheimer's Community Care, West Palm Beach, Florida
Sixteen-year caregiver for his wife, Jeannette

To learn more go to www.AlzheimersCareConsultants.com.

Caregiving Just got easier! 6/11
WARM wishes,
Nately

ALZHEIMER'S DISEASE AND OTHER DEMENTIAS

The Caregiver's Complete Survival Guide

ALZHEIMER'S DISEASE AND OTHER DEMENTIAS

The Caregiver's Complete Survival Guide

NATALY RUBINSTEIN

MSW, LCSW, C-ASWCM

Two Harbors Press
Minneapolis, MN

Two Harbors Press
212 3rd Avenue North, Suite 290
Minneapolis, MN 55401
612.455.2293
www.TwoHarborsPress.com

Author's Note

This publication is designed to provide accurate and authoritative information in regard to the subject matter covered. It is sold with the understanding that neither the publisher nor the author is engaged in rendering psychological, financial, legal, or other professional services. This work expresses the author's opinions and experiences and is not intended to provide and does not provide either psychological or medical advice. This book is not a substitute for your doctor. If expert assistance or counseling is needed, the services of a competent professional should be sought. Individual readers are solely responsible for their own health care decisions; the author and the publisher do not accept responsibility or liability for any adverse effects individuals may claim to experience, whether directly or indirectly, from the information contained in this book.

ISBN-13: 978-1-936198-13-9
LCCN: 2010941406

Distributed by Itasca Books

Cover Design by Wes Moore
Typeset by Sophie Chi

Printed in the United States of America

To my mother, Catherine:
Caring for you made me a better person.

CONTENTS

FOREWORD

We have come a long way in the fight against Alzheimer's disease and related dementias. Twenty years ago, when my uncle Bob was first diagnosed with Alzheimer's, there were no treatments. However, thanks to the help of science and medicine, we now have a variety of effective therapies that both patients and physicians can turn to.

There is no magic bullet in terms of treatment, especially for Alzheimer's, the most common form of dementia. Physicians must utilize a comprehensive approach of pharmacologic (e.g., FDA-approved drugs, medical food, supplements) and non-pharmacologic (e.g., physical exercise, mental exercise, music therapy for memory) means to provide optimal patient care.

Among the most vital of these non-pharmacologic interventions are education and caregiver support. I urge my patients, and especially their caregivers, to get educated about the disease. In my practice, I have found that one of the most important and most effective management tools involves consultation with an experienced and well-trained health care professional who understands the disease from both the personal and the professional level. A well-informed caregiver can have a profound positive impact on the patient's quality of life and the psychosocial aspects of the disease. Over time, dedicated caregivers can acquire a set of skills and level of understanding that help streamline a well-coordinated and comprehensive plan of care.

In the following chapters, you will have the opportunity to read the words of Nataly Rubinstein, the most skilled clinical social worker and geriatric care manager specializing in dementia care I have had the opportunity to work with. Her words are heartfelt and real, comprehensive and precise, well-informed and well-researched. I have relied on Nataly throughout the duration of my practice to provide advice and guidance to my patients. She understands all aspects of the disease and has helped countless caregivers navigate through its complexities. Because of the multifaceted scope of dementia, and with the constraints of the health care system today, providing optimal care in the outpatient setting is challenging. This book can be used as a supplement to the efforts of not only caregivers but also nurses, social workers, physicians, and other members of the dementia care team.

As a neurologist specializing in Alzheimer's disease and related dementias, I have dedicated my professional career to helping patients and caregivers struggling with these conditions. Based on my own personal and professional experience, I want to convey my utmost respect and admiration for caregivers reading this book who struggle with the day-to-day challenges of caring for a person with dementia. I can honestly say that without your help and commitment, fighting dementia would be a battle nearly impossible to win. While it is unfortunate that resources like this book were not available to help in my uncle's care, I am encouraged that its publication will help families in the present and in the future.

Today, there is more hope than ever that with each passing day, science and medicine will come closer to finding that magic bullet we are all so desperately searching for. In the interim, I urge you to read this book, stay informed, maintain your strength, and hold your head up. We are all in this battle together, and it is a fight that we can and must win.

Richard S. Isaacson, M.D.
Vice Chair of Education
Director, Alzheimer's Division
Associate Professor of Clinical Neurology
University of Miami Miller School of Medicine

PREFACE

I can remember the moment as if it was yesterday, but actually it was 1994. My ninety-six-year-old father, my eighteen-month-old daughter, and I, sitting together in the neurologist's office, were told the devastating news that my mother had Alzheimer's disease. I remember hearing the diagnosis and going numb. As the doctor talked about the progression of the disease and the current medications that would reduce her difficult behaviors, my brain tuned out most things he said. I can still recall the doctor's voice, but none of his words. It seemed as if he talked for hours, but it was just a few minutes. Once the doctor said, "Alzheimer's," all I heard was "blah, blah, blah." All I could think about was that Mom was no longer Mom and would never be Mom again. At the moment of her diagnosis, I lost my mother. The neurologist took away my mother as I knew her, when he said to my father and me, "There is no cure, no medication to reverse her condition. She will live for five more years, become like a baby, need constant care, and will die." he explained that his office would send someone to assess the home and recommend improvements. But there was something that was never discussed during the appointment: the answers to two very important questions. How were we—my father, my siblings, and I—going to get through the next few years, and how could we make this a better time for Mom and our family?

The clinic sent over a physical therapist who told us the changes we would need to put into place to make the home safer. We pulled up the carpeting and locked the doors as recommended, but it didn't make my father's life or mine any better. Mom found other ways to escape. She resisted bathing and had moments that I wouldn't wish on my worst enemy. We were later advised that because of her difficult moments we should institutionalize her. When a person has dementia, they will have moments of clarity and still be capable of making choices. And make choices she did. Over the years, as I cared for her, I watched my mother move back and forth between childlike moments and coherent, rational moments. I never knew whom I was going to be dealing with. And after my father's death, my mother's care became my responsibility— my siblings walked away. At the time I didn't think I had any choice; her care had to become my priority.

There are more than 37 million people in the world who have dementia. Alzheimer's disease affects over 5 million people in the United States. It is the most known form of the eighty-six dementias and gets the most publicity. Maybe it is because some doctors automatically diagnosis any form of memory loss as Alzheimer's. There are other types of dementia that receive less press and are equally devastating to the person and their family. When you combine people who are affected by Lewy Body disease, Picks disease, frontal temporal dementia, vascular dementia, Parkinson's, and AIDS, and add in the number of people who have any form of memory loss the numbers will rise by millions more in the United States. People are getting diagnosed earlier and there are a large number who have mild cognitive impairment. This number does not include all of the people who are having memory loss and are undiagnosed or do not get an accurate diagnosis.

Statistics are just numbers. Until you personally know or have to deal with a person who has dementia, you won't know how being a caregiver will affect you. Your boss, friends, family, and relatives may acknowledge your situation and give you some form of support, but they may have no idea of the physical, emotional, and financial challenges you will face. At this time, you may not be prepared for these challenges yourself.

As a caregiver, you might wonder how you will be able to afford care for your loved one. Caring for a person with dementia will affect not only your current job but also your future career in terms of promotions, Social Security, pension, and health benefits. For those in the "sandwich" generation, caring for a person with dementia will affect your relationships with your children, spouse, and siblings as well as your emotional and financial relationships.

This book will help you, the caregiver, no matter what type of dementia you are dealing with, to get through this time successfully. As a licensed clinical social worker and geriatric care manager I worked with neurologists who specialize in dementia at the Wien Center at Mount Sinai Medical Center in Miami Beach, Florida, as well as neurologists within Mount Sinai and at the University of Miami. I know that when a person has any form of memory loss, it will change their life. Until a brain autopsy is performed, you cannot know for sure what type of dementia the person you are caring for has. When it comes to managing any form of memory loss, the diagnosis is just a tool. In the long run, knowing what type of dementia your loved one has is just a start on your caregiver journey. As the caregiver you will need to know how to deal with the person's memory loss, and the behavioral and personality changes that will happen. This book will guide you through this time of uncertainty in both of your lives.

When my mother was diagnosed with dementia, there were few books on the subject. What was written either didn't apply to my situation or left me without hope of caring for my mother's needs. The books that I read were confusing and depressing. Nothing addressed my current situation: the challenge of coping with my mother's behavioral changes and where to go for help. This book was written at the request of countless caregivers who have attended my workshops or whom I've met in my private practice. The caregivers I meet wanted to know why there is not one simple-to-read book that could help them. They found the information that I presented invaluable and kept after me to write all the information down so that other caregivers could benefit. I have heard from countless caregivers how much they would like to attend educational groups but for personal reasons could not. Clearly there is a need for some simple-to-understand tips and practical guidance for caregivers of people with memory loss.

This book is written for the person who wants to learn how to successfully care for a loved one with dementia. It is a practical guide that will give you valuable information about dementia and how to cope with its effects. You will learn how to deal with behavioral and emotional changes as well as how to get an accurate diagnosis, how to manage insurance, and how to locate resources. This book was written to address your concerns, answer your questions, and give you the direction and information that you will need to become a successful caregiver—it is your caregiver survival plan and will give you the information that you need and guide you through the actions that you will need to take at this time. I know that dealing with a person who has dementia at times can be difficult. Finding ways to help your loved one and you will from this point on be easier.

CHAPTER ONE

A BRIEF LOOK AT CAREGIVING

Lesson One: *How Did We Get Here?*

For many of us, it starts as little things that our loved ones now do or no longer do. Over time, you may notice that your loved one isn't acting "like their old self." Repetitive stories, misplaced items, and forgetting things like conversations, holidays, dinner plans, or a movie they saw recently signal that something isn't right. Your loved one may have trouble following the story line of a television show, a conversation, or a train of thought. You may find endless lists placed around the house or hear the excuse, "I've cooked my entire life, and now I don't want to anymore." Things that were once important seem to have lost their value. Hobbies are left by the wayside. Mom has stopped attending her weekly bridge game, or Dad has lost his interest in golf. What was once considered trash is now treasure. A family member may become obsessed with cutting coupons out of the newspaper or filling out sweepstake forms. Junk mail now becomes their most important correspondence because they now believe that they have just won a million dollars from a Clearing House Sweepstakes—and they know it is true because it says so on the envelope. You may notice that your loved one has become very generous and is freely giving away money or possessions to not only family members but total strangers who call them on the phone or knock on their door. Save the Whales, Save the Children, Save the Home—it doesn't matter: they just give when asked, and then forget they gave, and give again. Maybe you notice a change in personality. A normally calm person becomes increasingly angry, or an angry person becomes docile. And then there are some people who take on new personality traits that baffle us. Unexplained or unwarranted anger, secrecy, obsessive compulsiveness, paranoia, or inappropriate sexual behaviors occur out of nowhere. A personality change happens quickly—and then it's gone, and the person we care about is back to their old self, at least for now. Their new behavior is quickly explained as normal aging.

Many of the changes we accept as normal aging are not always normal. So what is normal? It's normal for couples who have been together for a while to finish each other's stories because these are their shared experiences. It's normal to call a family member by another person's name. It's normal to forget a doctor's appointment or a birthday because as we grow older, time and dates can lose their significance. A person can lose interest in their hobbies when their hobbies are too difficult to do because of physical changes—arthritis in their hands, knees, or back can make moving around difficult or painful. Some people stop doing a favorite activity because they no longer have someone with whom to share their interests. Friends and family move away or pass on. The person may no longer be able to drive to attend activities. Vision or hearing problems can also lead someone to discontinue a once-enjoyed activity. Mouth problems such as pain, missing teeth, or dentures can cause a person to withdraw socially because they're embarrassed to eat or speak in front of others.

What is not normal aging? Meals that are burned, undercooked, or forgotten after they were made or eaten. Dishes put in the dishwasher and then removed before the machine is turned on or soap added. You might begin to notice that some things are not where they are supposed to be. Food that should be in the refrigerator is now in the pantry. Dirty clothes are put in a garbage can instead of the hamper. A bucket in the garage is now being used as a toilet. If you ask questions about these things, you might hear reasonable responses such as, "I ran the dishwasher almost empty and decided to put a few more things in and run it again," or "I no longer want to wear those clothes so I threw them out," or "I couldn't make it to the bathroom, so I used what was handy." Some people may make light of these moments by saying, "Silly me, what was I thinking?" or "You know that I am so worried about your (father, mother, taxes, economy, etc.) that I can't think straight." When a person forgets an event, they might say, "Since I stopped working, the days aren't important" or "...my days fly by," which may at the time make perfect sense. You should know that any of these responses, no matter how normal or logical they may sound, are not a part of normal aging.

Dementia is not always about memory loss. For some people who are having memory loss, the first sign that they are having a problem may be a change in their behavior. Often a person who is having a memory problem will try to stick to a routine that they believe will keep them sane and at the same time keep their loved ones in the dark. The person that you care for may become obsessed with keeping to their routine. For a person with memory loss, structure becomes important. A person who is starting to have memory loss will cling to normalcy by having a daily routine that they now follow religiously. This gives a person with memory problems an illusion of control and an assurance that all is well.

As a caregiver, you should know that dementia will affect each person differently. When you meet one person with dementia, you have met just one person. Everyone is different, and how they compensate for memory loss will be different. Memory loss for each person is unique and will affect each person differently. When a person has memory loss, they may become more generous and freely donate money to various mail and phone solicitations for charities. They may become overgenerous with friends, relatives, and strangers. They may give away an admired article of clothing, a piece of jewelry, or a work of art to anyone who shows interest. Later in the day (or week or month), they may forget that they gave the item away and may have behavioral problems because they are now trying to locate this item. Some people can become miserly, or paranoid. A person who has memory loss is vulnerable. Because of their short-term memory loss and their need to appear normal, someone with memory loss is an easy target for unscrupulous people.

As a caregiver, you too are vulnerable. It doesn't matter whether you live far away, down the street, or in the same home; you may at first have no clue that a person is having trouble with their memory because most people with memory loss are brilliant conversationalists. Given the opportunity, they can and will talk endlessly about their day and life—as long as you do not ask for details. Even if you do ask specific questions, the person with memory loss will have a good recall of past events and then can quickly steer the conversation to a different topic.

Twenty-five years ago I was clueless about dementia. Nobody in my life (doctors, friends, family, or neighbors) talked about it or dealt with it. I lived a few miles away from my parents, whom I saw daily. I brought them dinners or took them out to eat and handled their finances. I was in constant communication with them. Every morning I spoke with my mom on the phone or later in the day saw her in person. Mom told me in detail what she had for breakfast and which restaurant she ate in. This gave me the assurance that everything at home was okay. I know that my mother can't cook; she is the only person I know who can burn water. Late in her life she discovered the breakfast menu at a local fast food restaurant and for the next several years was their best customer.

Every day I drove to my parents' home in the afternoon and spent four to five hours with them. I either picked up food for dinner or took them out to eat. One day I changed my routine and came over earlier. Mom was reading the newspaper in the same chair she had sat in for the last thirty years. She was in the same clothes she had on when I had seen her the day before. I casually asked her if she had had breakfast. Mom told me where she went, what she ate, and how delicious the meal was. At this time, a red flag came up. There was no way that my mother would ever leave the house without makeup or a clean outfit. I knew something was wrong and spoke with Dad about my concerns. Dad said that Mom hadn't left the house for breakfast for weeks, but he never said anything to me because he didn't want me to worry. Before that day, we had both sensed that something was wrong, but neither of us wanted to talk about or face what was happening.

This leads me to the subject of avoiding a situation, also known as denial. Denial is a natural response that we use to avoid an unwanted, undesired, or unexpected situation. It is normal to think that if we deny what is happening, the situation will stop, reverse itself, or not occur at all. If I don't acknowledge a problem, the problem doesn't exist. If I ignore a problem, it will go away. By not acknowledging that there is a problem, I ensure that my world will remain the same—life as I know it will continue, and the reality of what is happening will disappear. Denial serves a personal purpose. Many of us may go into a state of denial because the new information that is presented is overwhelming, and our brain naturally shuts down. This is a normal protective mode for personal survival. Eventually, there will come a time when you will have to deal with the reality of the situation, but at this time you are not able to. You might go into the denial mode because you do not want to take on the additional responsibility of care for a person with dementia. Fear and grief are a normal part of denial. I often refer to denial as voluntary self-deception. The reality is, at some point, you will recognize that there is a "now" situation that needs to be addressed.

There will come a time when your loved one who has dementia will need additional help from you or from others to make it through their day. The help you give will change the dynamics of your relationship. How you view your relationship with your loved one may change the moment that they are diagnosed. Your new role of being a caregiver may change not only your relationship with the person you are caring for but all your relationships. Unlike many other diseases, dementia has no cure or timeline. There are no medications that can stop or reverse this disorder, although some treatments and therapies can slow it down. There are three key things you can do to improve your life and the life of the person with memory loss: education, accurate diagnosis, and action.

Lesson Two: *No Two Dementias Are Alike*

If I had a dollar for each time I heard someone say, "I know all about dementia; my (mother, father, aunt, uncle, grandmother, grandfather, mother-in-law, father-in-law, cousin, and /or neighbor) had dementia, and I know all about it," I could retire with a little help from my financial planner. The reality is that each time I hear those words, I cringe. Just because I have two teenage children does not by any means make me an expert on teenagers. It just makes me an expert on the two teenagers who live with me. And as anyone who has teenagers will tell you, they are all unique and constantly changing, as is the relationship I have with them. Between their wants and needs and my own, I have become a circus juggler. On a daily basis I have what seems like ten balls in the air. To keep them all up in the air, I need to adapt to their world. Each moment of my life is a compromise. Teenagers, like toddlers, are totally self-centered; the entire world revolves around them. This same understanding applies to a person with dementia.

My kids, a boy and a girl, were born six years apart. They have different life experiences, different goals, different habits, and different needs. I was a different person when I started parenting my son from who I was when my daughter was born. For me to treat them the same because they are now both teenagers would disregard who they are as individuals and their own special needs. This is no different for the person who has dementia. Each person is unique and should be treated as such. If you use what worked for one person on another person, the result might not be successful. What calms one person may cause unwanted or aggressive behaviors in another. Every person's personality is different. I have met some people with dementia who are the happiest people on earth, who love to laugh and smile, and I have met others whose behaviors are so difficult that even Mother Teresa would find them challenging to deal with.

Every day we have an opportunity to learn, grow, and change our thoughts about a situation or our behavior. We are constantly changing, evolving, and reestablishing new behaviors. New information gives us an opportunity to change the way we deal with any situation. Over time, working, caring for our families, interacting and reacting to current events will change us. As adults we bring to our world a bundle of emotions—hopes and dreams, disappointments, fears, and insecurities—as well as our life experiences that have made us who we are today. What we do and how we react are based on past experiences. Memory is highly individual and personal. Memories are elusive and subjective. What this means is that your recall of a situation is based on you. Your perception of any event is now your reality. Most of our memories are based on the intensity of our current emotions and our recall of the past. The past is a funny thing. Your view of the past may change over time to make memories better or worse, depending on what outcome you want. Memories are often only as good or as bad as you want them to be to justify your actions in the present. Things might not have gone the way you wanted as a child or spouse or caregiver, and still today you continue to judge, act, and react based on your recall of these moments. This is where many behavior problems start.

From the moment you choose or are chosen by the family to become a caregiver, you need to understand that memory loss, which is under the umbrella of dementia, is the great equalizer. People with dementia are no longer able to be responsible for many of their words or actions. People with dementia have a personal freedom. On the outside, a person will look, act, and speak like an adult, and at the same time they connect with their inner emotional child. Their social mask is now off. For them, there is no awareness of the future; the person you care about is living in the "now."

When a person has dementia, what you see is what you get. At some point during this disorder, you will meet and experience your loved one as they truly are. Prepare yourself: this person you thought you knew so well may surprise you. At times they will behave like an infant, toddler, or teenager: totally self-absorbed. Because their brain has changed and will continue to change, a person with dementia is no longer capable of controlling their impulses. You are dealing with a person who is no longer constrained by social rules. To successfully deal with the person with memory loss, you will have to let go of what worked or what you think may have worked for you or someone else in the past.

Caring for a person with memory loss is not easy. Actually, there are times when it may be downright difficult. The relationship you have with this person will change, and the changes will affect your life. The reality is that caring for a person with dementia will take a financial, social, and emotional toll on you.

Lesson Three: *Who Is a Caregiver?*

Everyone who cares for another person is a caregiver. In my practice, I deal with over eight hundred clients a year. From my years working at Mount Sinai and my private practice, I have met thousands of families. This book was written and rewritten several times. Depending on the audience I was writing for, one form of the book was helpful to the professional or the caregiver, two different audiences with similar yet different ways of approaching dementia. On my computer I have four almost complete forms of this book, each written with a different style and information. One addressed the needs of professionals, another was geared to institutions, another was for caregivers, and the fourth was additional tips gathered over my twenty-five years in the field. All four books would stand on their own, but something about each of them felt incomplete. As a writer, therapist, and caregiver I was stuck on what direction this book should take. And then I met Sam.

Sam brought his ninety-two-year-old mother to our center after she was diagnosed by another doctor two weeks previously with Alzheimer's disease. Their doctor had told Sam that if his mother did not take the medication he prescribed, "She will be a child in one year." Sam told me that since the day he had heard those words, he had experienced the worst two weeks of his life. I spent the next hour and a half giving Sam and his mother a crash course on dementia—the disease, the stages, medication, and alternative therapies—and I suggested several activities that might help his mother retain her current abilities for a longer period of time. I also explained the importance of diet, exercise, and proper hydration. Based on her current needs, we discussed hiring a paid companion. When they left my office, Sam hugged me and thanked me for the diagnosis. I was floored: I never gave a diagnosis. His mother definitely had short-term memory loss. I gently reminded Sam that I hadn't given them a diagnosis. "Oh yes you did," he said. "You gave us the diagnosis of hope."

It dawned on me that what was missing in my previous drafts of this book was a focus on what caregivers of people with dementia have in common. All of us are caregivers. The doctors, nurses, social workers, day care workers, spouses, children, in-laws, friends, neighbors, and volunteers have huge roles in the care of a person with dementia and their family. To be a good doctor it is no longer enough to diagnose this disorder; they must take into account what the diagnosis will mean to the family. Nurses need to understand how this disease is going to affect the individual and to explain the medication that will be needed to deal with the changes. Social workers need to understand this disease, the impact it will have on the family, and the potential behavioral changes, and they need to be able to recommend community resources. Day care workers and home health aides need to know how to recognize the different stages of this disorder to be better able to interact in meaningful activities. Family members for a person who has dementia will need all of this information and more; they will need hands-on-deck, custom-designed guidance that combines their needs and the needs of the person with memory loss.

Above all, everyone needs hope. Not a hope for a speedy cure or a miracle pill that will return all of our lives to normal, but rather for a way to deal with dementia with dignity for all concerned. As our lives change as caregivers, we hope to find the ability to reshape our dreams and maintain our quality of life. Hope like this comes from having good tools to be the best caregivers we can be.

Many caregivers are experts in their field. The doctors, lawyers, nurses, accountants, and business owners I help are the "master of their universe" in their jobs, but when it comes to dealing with dementia in their own homes, they are just as confused about how to deal with dementia as you are. I'm sure you've heard the expression "It's not rocket science." Some of my caregiver clients actually worked for NASA—they are rocket scientists! They have put people on the moon, but they have no idea how to deal with a person who has dementia on Earth. The same goes for caregivers who are doctors or nurses. Many of these caregivers are successful in their specific fields, but they are only experts in their one field. Toss in a diagnosis of dementia, and they are no different from anyone else. Some of my caregiver clients are neurologists; when it comes to dealing with their own family members, they have an understanding about the changes in the brain, but they are at a loss as to how to deal with the behavioral issues that result.

There is no "one size fits all" when you are dealing with a person who has dementia. You are unique; your relationship with this person is one of a kind; the person you are dealing with is like no other. Remember that you are human. Many of us have a working life and additional responsibilities besides caring for a person with memory problems. In order to be a successful caregiver you will need to have a good team in place. You cannot care for a person with dementia alone.

To be a successful caregiver, there will be times you will have to inhale deeply, exhale, and then seek support. When I first started writing this book, I was a graduate student working with elders at a large local nursing home. I completed my internship at the Wien Center, which at that time had two licensed clinical social workers. Over the past several years, because of circumstances, at times I was the only social worker on staff. My job is to help families deal with the diagnosis of dementia. Some of the families I see are Hispanic, and even though I understand Spanish, speaking their language, depending on the region that they come from, is a challenge. I arrive home exhausted. I also have a private practice. When I walk out of either office, I am a caregiver to my mother, who has dementia, as well as a mom to two children who are now teenagers. I am lucky: over the years I have developed and nourished a good support system. I have friends I can depend on to pick up my children from school when I'm not able to. I also work close to home and live in the neighborhood of my children's schools, which gives me the flexibility to pick up a sick child or take them to an after-school activity and be back in my office in less than fifteen minutes. I can also get home to care for my mother in five minutes. My job is 2.4 miles from my home. This sounds like a luxury, but I pay for it financially. The facility that I work for pays less for my services than other jobs that are further away.

Caregiving is a trade-off. When it comes to dealing with my mother, all bets are off, and her care is mine alone. Family and friends are sometimes unavailable; my mother is my responsibility. I know from experience that caring for a person with a memory disorder can be physically, emotionally, and financially draining.

Lesson Four: *Know Thyself*

As a caregiver, it is important to understand yourself before you begin to care for a loved one with memory loss. For potential caregivers I call this the "who, why, what, when, where, and how" moments. Before you sign on to be a caregiver, you should think long and hard about yourself and your situation. When the going gets rough, you need to keep in mind the reasons you have chosen to take on this new responsibility, and these reasons will provide you comfort. If you answer the questions below honestly, you will be doing yourself and the person you are caring for a huge favor. If you lie to yourself, you may end up feeling resentful, regretful, frustrated, and burdened. Be realistic. Over time you will change, the person you are caring for will change, and your situation may change. Remember, nothing is set in stone.

1. WHO is the person you will be caring for? Are they your spouse, parent, sibling, grandparent, close or distant relative, in-law, friend, or neighbor? How is your relationship with them now? What was it like in the past? Not everybody has a good relationship with family members. Being a caregiver means you will now be in charge. This role reversal is difficult no matter whom you are caring for. If your husband has always made all of the decisions, it may be hard for you to start taking charge. Many children have a difficult time in learning how to be a parent to their parent.

2. WHY are you choosing to be a caregiver? There are many reasons a person chooses to become a caregiver.

Be honest with yourself. Are you doing this out of love or because you feel a sense of obligation? Is it because you live closer to the person than other family members, or do you have a better relationship with the person you are going to care for? Are you getting back at the person for past mistreatment or trying to fulfill a dream of the perfect relationship? Some people use their caregiver position for financial gain, while some may see it as an opportunity to escape from their current adult responsibilities and now have an excuse to withdraw from living their life.

3. WHAT are you dealing with? Knowledge is power. Has the person you will now be caring for had a proper diagnosis? Realize that the care a person with dementia will need can span from this moment to possibly twenty years or more. To get you through this time you will need to have a firm understanding of this disorder. As a caregiver, you will need not only to understand this disease but to continually seek out additional resources such as support groups, educational programs, community resources, and respite services. To be a successful caregiver, you will need to know the type and stage of dementia the person has now and be prepared for what might happen in the future as the disorder progresses.

4. WHEN do you need to provide care? In the early stage of dementia, the care needed is usually easy to give. A kind word, a simple suggestion, a phone call, or a visit is all that both of you may now need. Over time, as this disorder progresses, you may need to provide more care—from supervision to actual hands-on care.

The more care that is needed, the more it will affect you physically, financially, and emotionally.

5. WHERE are you going to provide the care? Depending on the level of care required, some caregivers may make a decision to either move in with the person who has memory loss or relocate this person into their home. Do you have the space, or are you willing to add to your home? Before making any decision you should take your job, relationships, and daily life into consideration. If you live in another part of town or out of state, consider hiring a geriatric care manager to help you make a good decision as to what resources will be needed that will allow the person to remain where they are now or to recommend a facility that will be appropriate and will provide for better care.

6. HOW will you make this work? There is no simple answer. I wrote this book to give you the tools you will need and guide you through this new situation. There is no "one size fits all" when it comes to caregiving. What works for one person may not work for you. You are unique, your situation and relationship are unique, and the person you are caring for is unique. Overtime, as a caregiver you too will change, and your life and needs as well as the person you are caring for will change. You will need to keep an open mind and be patient.

Being a caregiver is not for everyone. If you feel anger or animosity, despite your good intentions you might not be the best person for this job. Be honest about how you feel about the person, and know why you choose to care for them. In the long run, you may need to do what is best for you and for them. Not everyone is cut out to be a caregiver for a person who has dementia. As a potential caregiver, you need to know that there will come a point in time that you will need additional assistance to help you care for your loved one. Caring for a person with dementia is not something that in the long run, you can do alone.

There is no one right way to caregiving—we all follow our own path. Each of us has our own style. No matter what road you take, understanding how the brain is affected and changing over time because of this disorder is important. Learning about medication, behavioral techniques, community resources, and governmental and private-pay insurance plans will help you deal with this situation. Education is power. The more you know about dementia, the better caregiver you will be.

CHAPTER TWO

UNDERSTANDING DEMENTIA

To handle this new situation you have found yourself in, you will need to have some basic understanding of what you are dealing with. Remember that when you meet one person with dementia, you have met just one person with dementia. No two dementias are the same. Each person will travel on their own road. Each road will be different because of their unique lifestyle, environment, genetics, character, and personality and the course of their disorder. When it comes to dealing with a person who has dementia, the most important component is you, the caregiver. The relationship you have with your loved one, be it as a spouse, child, friend, neighbor, or paid companion, will have a dramatic effect on how this disorder evolves. You can't deal with what you don't know. Understanding this disorder will help you cope and give you the tools to care for the person with dementia the best way possible.

Lesson One: *Understanding the Brain*

What can I say but, "Welcome to your brain!" To better understand and deal with dementia you will need to understand a little bit about how the brain works. Researchers who study the brain are publishing new information every day. The more they know, the less they used to know. For now, this is what we know.

Our brain is the most miraculous organ we have. Unfortunately, it is also the most taken for granted, unknown, and least understood of all our body parts. Sitting within our skull, hidden from view, is our life force. Everything we do or don't do is ruled by the brain. The brain regulates everything that occurs in our bodies: our thoughts, memories, and actions as well as the functions of all of our internal organs. Our heart, kidneys, blood flow, liver, lungs, bladder, and bowels (to name just a few) are all regulated by the brain. You just blinked, sighed, coughed, yawned, swallowed, took in a breath, or turned a page; this is all controlled through your brain. Every conscious and unconscious thought, action, and emotion are products of our brain. The brain sends out millions of signals a day that keep us functioning and allow us to continue to survive. When the brain stops sending signals to the rest of the body, we stop functioning.

Most of us go about our lives without giving any thought to our brains. We take our actions and thoughts for granted because our brains allow us to. We only have one brain. The brain doesn't come in pairs like other organs such as eyes, ears, legs, or kidneys. Unlike other organs such as the heart, liver, or lungs, the brain cannot be replaced. There are no skin grafts, prosthetics, or donor that can replace your brain. Your brain is one of a kind: it not only regulates your body's daily functions but is filled with your personal life—your experiences, emotions, dreams, hopes, aspirations, and memories. Your brain is you.

Protected and hidden by bones and covered by skin and hair is the one organ that controls all you are. The brain is like an incredible computer. It takes in and stores all of your life experiences from the time you were conceived up until today. The brain is a remarkable record keeper. Life experiences such as abuse, neglect, trauma, and war will affect the brain. Alcohol, smoking, drugs, food, and even the environment- like lead paint exposure or pesticides will affect the newly forming brain as well as an adult brain. Past and current jobs, relationships, and lifestyle will affect the brain. Nutrition will affect the brain. Stress will affect the brain, and so will depression. The way you learn is shaped by your brain. Even your relationships are shaped by your brain. According to current science, nature supplies billions of neurons in the brain of a developing fetus, but thousands of these neurons are lost after birth because they are no longer used. We have more neurons at birth than we do as an adult!

A mere one and a half quarts in volume, or approximately three pounds, the mass that sustains and drives us is packed with 100 billion cells, which include 10,000 synapses with 100 trillion connections that contain 300 million feet of wiring. Cells are arranged in six different layers that allow the brain's regions to carry out vision, hearing, sensation, balance, smell, and movement as well as to regulate all other organs.

For now, science has divided the brain into different sections. Each section has a role. There are areas of the brain responsible for speech, memory, movement, smell, and life. The brain allows us to live our life on autopilot. The brain controls being what is automatically done, and controls for everything that we do—physically, emotionally and mentally. The brain is composed of axons, dendrites, and neurons that connect and communicate to one another. A neuron is a brain cell, and we are born with 100 billion of them. We also have neurotransmitters as well as a host of chemicals produced naturally in the brain, such as norepinephrine (fixes information into long-term memory), endorphins (brain morphine), serotonin (depression/sleep and relaxation), GABA (behavior), and acetylcholine (REM sleep). What is important to keep in mind is that the brain is constantly changing. As a caregiver, you need to remember that every person's brain is unique but all brains need a certain amount of naturally produced chemicals to keep a person functioning properly. If the brain produces less of these chemicals, memory and personality will change. Science and drug companies have developed medications that are used to compensate for these losses, although medications work differently for each individual.

The brain is designed to work on autopilot. This simply means that many of the things we normally do occur without any thought or purpose from us. The brain is self-regulating. Take breathing, for example. You don't think about breathing (unless you have asthma, just walked up a flight of stairs, or are using an oxygen tank); it just naturally happens. In short, this automatic thing that the brain does allows us to live and to go through our day easily. I could go on for hours about what the brain does, but for now, let's focus on memory and dementia.

The brain remembers and recalls everything and every moment of what we have done or want to do. Forget the family photo album—the brain has a memory of its own. The brain records semantic memory, which is the retention of facts, language, and knowledge as well as procedural knowledge that involves skills. Episodic memory—our personal timeline—connects us to our selves. The brain records everything that we have ever done, learned, or thought.

As of now, science believes that the brain is divided into sections, each of which has a specific job. The frontal lobe is responsible for planning, organizing, personality and behavior, emotions, speech, motor skills, and conscious thought. The parietal lobe processes sensory input and body orientation. The occipital lobe is responsible for visual reception and interpretation. The temporal lobe is where language is processed. The cerebellum coordinates body movements, and the corpus callosum connects both of the hemispheres of the brain. The right side of the brain controls visual skills, and the left side of the brain controls logic and reasoning. Certain sections determine what information needs to reach these areas and other parts, such as the hypothalamus and the pituitary gland, which controls growth, sex, and the body's "clock." In summary, different areas of the brain control different functions. Here is where it gets tricky; the brain stores memories in more than just one area, and this will affect how your loved one's memories are stored and recalled. If the brain is damaged in one area, other parts of the brain may take over to help the damaged area. If this confuses you, you are in good company: scientists still do not understand how the brain functions.

What we do know is that because of changes to their brain, a person with dementia will at some point have difficulty in the use of language (talking), comprehension (understanding), judgment (decisions), and coordination (walking and/or manual skills). This will change how they deal with life. Learned skills such as driving, cooking, bathing, and using the remote control for the television eventually will diminish over time. There may come a point when the person with dementia will become confused by people and situations. Their current recollection of events may blend their past memory with the present and may include imagined moments. Over time, a person with dementia will have problems understanding what they need to do as well as what they want to do. Episodic memory is our personal timeline; when memory loss occurs, we will forget dates or specific facts from our episodic memory. Events blur, timelines intersect, and memories may no longer be accurate.

Until recently, it was considered scientific fact that memory was stored in one specific area of the brain. If this area of the brain was damaged or destroyed, scientist believed that the person's memories were lost forever. It has been recently discovered that memories may be retrieved from different areas of the brain, and even if one part of the brain is damaged, over time another area of the brain may be able to compensate for the damaged part.

Everyday, new things are discovered about the brain. Up until 2005, it was believed that once a neuron died, it was lost; in 2006, we learned that no matter what the age of the person, new neurons develop every day. In 2007, researchers discovered that brain cells communicate with their "neighbors" and that neurons work together, which may account for how memory can be retrieved. Despite scientific advancement, the brain is still a complex mystery. The brain's wiring is unique and intricate, and when you add to the mix the role that the environment plays, the brain becomes even harder to understand. Science is not perfect or all-knowing.

Lesson Two: *What Is Dementia?*

Dementia is a syndrome of intellectual impairment that is irreversible and progressive. Dementia affects a person's memory, judgment, reasoning, comprehension, logic, and recall. What this means to you, the caregiver, is that there is now a loss of mental function in the person you care for, and over time they will need more help from you or another person to remain independent.

Some people who have memory loss are still able to understand and comprehend what is happening to them; others fight these changes. It doesn't matter how a person performs on a neurocognitive test, or their diagnostic outcome, what is important to know is that every person continues to be an individual. They had a life before the diagnosis, and they should be able to continue to have a purposeful life after the diagnosis. A person who has dementia is above all a human being. They deserve to be treated with dignity and respect throughout their life.

As a caregiver you need to be aware that for those who are having memory problems in the beginning and middle stages of dementia, memory loss is not total; some areas of the brain may work well, while others do not. This can be frustrating and distressing to the person with dementia and to the caregiver. A person with dementia may have many moments of clarity, especially when it comes to activities they have always done. Sometimes a person with dementia can remember things and will be able to do them well, while other memories and skills seem to slip away. One moment they are "with it," and the next moment they are not. Caregivers often get frustrated by this "light switch" change in memory. They tell me, "At home he barely talks to me, but when we go out, I can't shut him up," or "She asks me the same question a hundred times a day, but when the kids come over, she never repeats questions to them."

Many caregivers believe that what their loved one may say or do is done to purposefully annoy them. Trust me: this is not the case. A person who is having memory loss, because of changes to their brain, will have times when the connections in their brain work well, and then, like a light switch that turns off and on, they will lose the ability to process information. A person with dementia will also have moments when they just shut down. As a caregiver, you will need to understand that certain regions of the brain are being affected by this disorder, and other areas of the brain are functioning normally. When a person has memory loss, some skills may be impaired or lost, but there are still areas of their brain that are not affected, so there are things they are still able to do—and do well.

The average person with dementia goes through three main stages over two to fifteen years. (I say "average" because there are extremes. I have seen some people decline within nine months and pass away, and I know others who are still alive after twenty-two years.) Each person will have some decline, although the actual rate of decline will be different for each individual. Within the three main stages—mild, moderate, and severe—there are several sub stages. Because each person is unique, the progress of dementia will vary. For some people, their memory loss will be like a spiral; others may have a step-like memory loss; and then there are those who will have a steep downward memory decline. If the person you are caring for has a sudden onset of memory loss, it may be due to a medical problem (such as a stroke, dehydration, or a urinary tract infection) and is often reversible. A step-like progression is when all appears good and then suddenly there is a downward change: the person with dementia seems to go over a cliff, and then all is well for a while until they go over the next cliff. A steep decline can be caused by a medical or environmental condition such as a change in medication or a change in their home life.

For many of my clients, the progression of memory loss is gradual. Rarely does a person have a steady downward decline. It is more like a spiral, similar to a tornado or water spout. At times, the person with memory loss seems normal, and then later on, whether it is minutes or hours later, they seem totally normal, like their old self. During the course of the day, they go between knowing what is going on around them, having some awareness, and having no clue, and then they have periods of time where they are back to their old self.

For some people, memory loss can be a normal part of their aging, however for others, memory loss and dementia is a serious form of memory loss that interferes with the way a person thinks, talks, and acts. On my office desk I have a poster that I use to help families understand dementia. Once they see the poster and understand the changes in the brain, they have a better understanding of what is happening in and to the brain of the person who has dementia. Since you, the reader, can't see the poster, I want you to interlock your fingers with both hands to form a tight fist. Keep your fingers tight: this is your current brain. Now, slowly start to open your hands; the greater the space between your fingers, the harder it is for the neurotransmitters to connect with each other and communicate among themselves. Keep spreading your fingers. As the gaps widen, brain messages have a greater difficulty being sent or received because the wider the gap, the harder it is to transmit and recall information. This is the brain of a person who has dementia.

Another way to explain dementia is to picture your brain as a road map. You know all the streets, exits, and side streets by heart. If there is a detour, roadblock, or heavy traffic, you know where to go and what you need to do to reach your destination quickly. When you have mild dementia, the road block (known as "plaques and tangles") will pose some problems, but eventually you will find a way around and reach your destination. When you have moderate dementia, the road blocks will cause more difficulty. The roads that you were once familiar with are now closed, and to get where you want to go is difficult and confusing. You may have to go down a few unfamiliar streets and take some turns before you find a road that will get you back to where you want to be. This will take time. When you have severe dementia, the road blocks will stop you. The road blocks are so complete that no matter which way you turn, you will get stuck at a dead end. There is no way out: there is nowhere to go; there is no safe turn. When a person has severe dementia, the plaques and tangles have taken over their brain, altering and stopping all communication. Their brain is on a form of autopilot; they can no longer draw information from the road map of their past nor design a new road map to get them through the day, to where they or you want them to be.

A person who has dementia survives by drawing on past memories that they can still recall and using their inner instinct to guide them. What they are doing may not make sense to you, but for them it makes total sense. As a caregiver, think of how you would feel going to a new place and being unsure of the road. You might feel scared, agitated, worried, or confused. This is how the person who has dementia feels, and it could be the reason why they might prefer to remain in bed or stay in their home.

For many of my clients, the idea of plaques and tangles in the brain and how they affect memory is difficult to understand. It was hard for me too, until I nicknamed the substance of plaques and tangles as "gunk." For me "gunk" is a green, mucus-type substance. I hear it as soft squishy noise. It feels sticky, like a piece of unwanted gum I accidentally stepped on with my shoe and I'm trying to get off. As we age, "gunk" is a substance that slows down and may even close down brain connections over time. I say "may" because science is no longer sure if the plaques and tangles are the cause of memory problems. There have been many cases in which people had no reported memory problems during their life, but after death, during the autopsy it is discovered that their brains were filled with plaques and tangles, while other people who had reported memory problems had no plaques or tangles.

Science is still learning about the brain. But for now the current belief is that the more gunk in the brain, the less a person can do, or the harder it will be to do what they once did. A diagnosis of dementia means that it will be difficult to learn new things, and over time it will be harder to remember previously learned things. A person with dementia will forget learned things. Their memories of events, people, and how to do activities they once learned and enjoyed will slowly become harder to retrieve and, in time, will eventually be forgotten.

Lesson Three: *Conditions that Mimic Dementia*

As you will see in the next chapter, many doctors incorrectly diagnosis dementia. Just because a person has memory loss doesn't mean that they have dementia. One of the first steps every doctor should take before diagnosing dementia is to rule out any condition that can mimic dementia or be the cause of memory loss. When properly treated, there are some forms of memory loss that can be reversed or reduced. The following are a few conditions that can cause or mimic memory loss and may be reversible if treated:

- depression
- hypothyroidism
- vitamin B-12 deficiency
- hydrocephalus
- neurosyphilis
- AIDS
- stroke
- alcoholism
- medication reaction
- brain tumor
- dehydration

- infection
- hypoglycemia/Diabetes
- liver failure
- vision loss
- hearing loss
- stress
- sleep disorder
- copper deficiency

The goal of a medical evaluation is to avoid a wrong diagnosis. If a person has memory loss from an undiagnosed brain tumor or thyroid malfunction, memory medication may be prescribed, but this is not going to help them. In later chapters, I will show you how some of these conditions can contribute to memory loss, but for now I will focus on just three from this list: depression, stress, and medication reaction.

Depression affects a person both emotionally and physically. In MRI brain scans, the person who is depressed will have a shrunken hippocampus (an area of the brain that looks like a horseshoe) like a person with dementia. A person who is depressed may socially withdraw, be apathetic, sleep too little or too much, eat too little or too much, cry, or feel like a burden, and some may think about ending their lives. A person who is depressed is in physical and emotional pain, which will affect their memory.

When you are in emotional pain, you withdraw and just focus on yourself. You will not care what day it is, not find a reason to get out of bed, and not want to bathe, eat, or answer the phone. When you are depressed, you really do not care about what happens in the outside world or even in your personal space. You will not pick up the phone to call friends or family; you will lose interest in current events and repeat the same conversations because you just want to get through the moment so that you will be left alone and can go back to bed. Family members become concerned because a depressed person seems forgetful and repetitive and is no longer caring for themselves. At the clinic where I worked, many of our new clients have untreated depression that has been misdiagnosed as dementia by family or other doctor.

For many years, I believed that stress is a major factor in memory loss. Over the past several years, I have had several discussions—actually, heated debates—with neurologists and psychiatrists over the importance that stress plays in memory loss. If I can help my clients reduce their stress, their memories most often improve or remain stable. At the 2004 Philadelphia Conference on Alzheimer's disease and Dementia it was reported that stress can cause deterioration in a person with Alzheimer's disease. Stress can be debilitating, just like depression. Stress can cause forgetfulness, sleep and eating problems, and changes in activity and personality. Some people handle stress better than others do— or so they believe. Some people seem to thrive under stress until they are hit with a major heart attack, stroke, depression, or panic attack. Each person's ways of dealing with stress will be different. Some put on a happy face and keep on going. Obstacles are now challenges: it's an "I can handle anything" mentality. "Throw it at me, and I can deal with it" is their motto. Stress can cause a change in personality, and the person may become irritable or have angry outbursts that are out of character. Think "road rage" for this group. Since stress builds up slowly, many people never realize that they are under tremendous stress. When it comes to stress, the body either adapts or breaks down. Think of a heart attack or a nervous breakdown.

To best explain stress, let me tell you a fable I read when I was younger about the straw that broke the camel's back.

The owner of a camel would walk through the desert and collect straw to sell later at the market. Whenever he found some straw, he would pick up a piece and place it in a sack on the camel's back. A piece of straw is light in weight—barely noticeable to the camel. Piece by piece, the straw added up, and slowly the sack became heavier. The camel got used to the weight and continued walking on as its owner collected pieces of straw and placed them in the sack on its back. As they got closer to the city, where the owner was planning to sell the straw and envisioned future prosperity, he placed one more piece of straw on the camel's back. The camel collapsed. The owner never made it to the market.

The story of the straw that broke the camel's back is a lesson to us about how stress can break down a person with memory loss or their caregiver. Stress arises in bad situations such as a divorce, death, job loss, or an unwanted move. The fact is that even the happiest of times can cause stress: a change of job or role in the family, the birth of a child, moving, or a wedding is stressful. Our body and brain cannot distinguish between good stress and bad stress. It just registers as stress. Stress can break you. Stress can be a cause of memory loss.

Another cause of memory loss is medication—an often ignored cause, especially in people over fifty. For many people medication that is either prescribed by the doctor or taken over the counter (OTC) can cause unwanted memory loss. The use of OTC medication is often unreported because it is believed that if you can buy it off the shelf in the grocery, drugstore or health food store it doesn't count as medicine. Wrong thinking! As we age, some people have trouble sleeping and will use sleep aids that have the term "P.M." on the label. Many OTC cough and cold products can have side effects, so you should always check the ingredients. While scanning down the list of ingredients on the label, if you see any ingredient that has any form of "benzo"—known as benzodiazepines—you should be aware that they may cause memory loss. The same thing applies to vitamins, beverages, and supplements.

Keep in mind that the person that you are caring for may have more than one doctor, and they often visit several doctors and may not mention all of their current medications. They will complain of sleep problems or pain, and the doctor will write them a prescription without knowing about other medications or supplements that the person is taking. This may cause a problem with memory loss. You might think that the local pharmacist will see a pattern—wrong thinking again. Many of the elderly use several different pharmacies depending on the prescription and the doctor who writes it.

Another hidden problem that often goes unspoken and unaddressed is drug sharing. For example, Mom now uses the drug that was prescribed for Dad when he was having trouble sleeping. The dosage is based on his medical and physical condition, which is the correct dosage for him, but not for Mom. The medication may be too strong for her and is now causing memory loss. Another situation is when well-meaning friends or family members share their unused medication with others. Since the medication the person borrowed wasn't prescribed for them, it is forgotten and not reported on their current medication log. The same thing goes for homeopathic medicine, herbs, supplements, teas, and vitamins. Just because a product is labeled "natural" does not mean that it is safe. Many people suffer serious side effects because of "natural" or OTC medications that they thought were safe. Even if used alone, OTC products can have severe consequences.

Lesson Four: *Dementia and Daily Life*

Dementia is a progressive irreversible degenerative brain disorder. Over time, a person with dementia will lose their ability to learn new information and their capability to remember or recall previously learned information. There are over eighty-six different types of dementias. Each may at first present differently, but all of them involve some form of memory loss. Alzheimer's disease is the one we hear about the most. It is the most recognized, because it is what primary care physicians will frequently diagnose for any type of memory loss. To date, it is estimated that there are over 5 million people in the United States with Alzheimer's disease. There are other types of dementia that receive less press but are equally devastating to the person and their families. Your loved one could possibly have one of these.

"Alzheimer's" has become the new buzz word; it is now the popular generic term for any form of memory loss. If someone has memory loss, it is automatically assumed that it is Alzheimer's disease or a "senior moment." For many doctors, memory loss is just that—memory loss. Some think that, based on a person's age, memory loss is a normal part of aging. Many doctors still believe that once you hit a certain age, your brain will automatically become forgetful. Nothing could be further from the truth. In reality, dementia comes in many forms: Vascular dementia, Lewy Body disease, Frontal Temporal disease, Parkinson's disease, Picks disease, and Creutzfeldt-Jakob disease, to name just a few. There is also AIDS-related dementia and dementias that are related to heavy metal and toxin exposure. Dementias can be caused by using or abusing prescription drugs, illegal drugs, and alcohol. On the other hand, just living life can be a cause of dementia: head trauma (a brain injury) can lead to dementia. Dementia is not always Alzheimer's disease, and different dementias will require different medication treatment.

Dementia affects speech, coordination, personality, behavior, and memory. Overtime, people who have dementia will lose their current ability to perform activities on their own and will need some outside assistance to help them successfully accomplish their activities of daily living (ADLs): grooming, bathing, eating, toileting, and moving around. Over time, the person with memory loss will lose their ability to do for themselves the normal activities also known as instrumental activities of daily living (IADLs), things that we typically do and take for granted, such as taking the correct dosage of medication, grocery shopping, balancing a checkbook, or planning a family outing or holiday dinner. A person with dementia will lose their ability to perform their IADLs before ADLs. ADLs are skills required for self-care: toileting, taking a shower or bath, dressing, eating a meal, or getting out of a chair. IADLs are those things that allow a person to live independently in the community (cooking, shopping, managing one's finances, etc.). Even though a person may still be able to dress themselves or go to the bathroom, if they are having difficulty shopping alone for food or can no longer work the stove or prepare a meal, then they no longer can live alone without some outside assistance.

Whether you live in the same house, next door, down the block, a few miles away, or states or continents away, one of the first signs that may alert you that something is not quite right is the loss of IADLs. Your loved one is now having trouble making plans, following through with doctor's appointments, or understanding directions. They may forget lunch dates, dinners, or special occasions. If a person is forgetting these important moments, can you really be sure they are taking their medication or eating right? The reality is that you can't be sure, and they probably aren't. A person with memory loss is no longer able to remember to take their medication by themselves. They can't remember what they have or haven't done. They may have difficulty shopping for food or clothing by themselves. A person with memory loss may have difficulty cooking or recognizing that food is spoiled. Often caregivers miss signs that additional care is needed. Most people with dementia will not ask for help because they want to remain independent. Some will not recognize that they need help.

A person with memory loss may repeat the same story several times or ask the same question for what seems like a hundred times, forget where they put things and then accuse you of stealing, keep detailed lists, hoard items, become paranoid, or become depressed. Some may become overly focused on sex, food (especially sweets), toileting, or money. Some will become overly friendly, while others may withdraw from family or friends.

As a caregiver, you need to keep in mind that dementia is a disorder of forgetting. Because of the changes in the brain, the person with dementia will lose their ability to remember things that most people take for granted. Looks can be deceiving: just because a person looks the same doesn't mean that they are capable of doing what they once did. Even though they may look the same, there will be times that they will lose their ability to distinguish what is proper or what is not. This is why they may now do or say things that are no longer considered socially acceptable. There will come a time when they no longer can figure out right from wrong or right from left. A person who is having memory problems may stubbornly insist on doing something their way, and as a caregiver you will cave in because you love them or no longer want to fight with them. When a person has dementia, present actions no longer hold future consequences. The present and the past become their "now." This very moment is their only reality. Their current wants, needs, hopes, desires, and thoughts all meld into the most basic primal urges as a form of survival or keeping to what is familiar. (Once again, think about a self-centered toddler or teenager.) As a caregiver in dealing with your loved one's new behaviors, you may be embarrassed, cringe, lash out, try to explain, or quietly accept what is going on, and/or you may withdraw from friends and family. Caring for a person with dementia will affect everyone in both of your lives.

There will come a time when the person with dementia will need your help to get through their day. You need to know that the care you provide will affect your relationships with family and friends, your career, your finances, and your future. As the person you are caring for slips further into dementia, the level of care they need will increase over time, and so will your responsibility. At some point you will have difficult choices to make. As a caregiver, you may value the care of your loved one over your own needs. The road of the caregiver is not easy.

For a person with dementia, maintaining their personhood is the key to helping them to remain physically and emotionally connected to their world. Every moment of maintaining their life is now an inward struggle and an outward fight for survival. They want to be understood, accepted, and acknowledged as a human being and to be respected for their role in the family and for their accomplishments. Every person deserves to be heard—no matter how loud or soft their voice may be. Life will go on despite dementia. No matter what form of memory loss a person has, they are still a viable, productive person even though they are trapped within the plaques and tangles of their brain.

Lesson Five: *Making Life Better for You and the Person with Dementia*

There are three keys to improving your life as a caregiver and the life of the person with memory loss: education, accurate diagnosis, and action.

Education is what you have begun from the moment you picked up this book. Each page is a learning opportunity. Through this book you will gain a wealth of knowledge about this disorder, and by the time you finish this book, you will be better equipped to understand yourself, dementia, and the person you care for. You will also have a number of resources to help you further.

Recent studies have shown that an educated caregiver can postpone assisted living or nursing home placement of a person with dementia by eighteen months. For many families, this means saving many dollars per year. I live in Miami Beach, Florida, where a good assisted living facility for dementia costs over $3,800 per month. This translates to an average cost of over $63,000 per year. I say "average" because if a person needs additional care, which they will over time, such as my mom in her current stage, the price dramatically goes up. If I placed my mom in a nursing home, I would pay $6,000 per month for a shared room; the total annual nursing home cost would be $72,000. This does not include the additional aides I would need to hire to make sure that she is well cared for.

An accurate diagnosis is essential to understanding this disorder. In the next two chapters you will learn about things to look for and ask for and what to expect from a doctor. You will learn how the medical and pharmaceutical companies work and how to use this information to help you and the person with memory loss.

Once you have the knowledge of this disorder combined with an accurate diagnosis, reading this book will give you most of the information you will need to deal with this disease. It will be the actions you choose to take that will bring it all together and help make all of this information work. I can guide you through the importance of an accurate diagnosis, prepare you to deal with difficult behaviors, inform you of the importance of respite and financial documents, and explain how to choose a care facility, but the rest will be up to you. Your actions will set the stage for how you handle this disorder and how this disorder will affect you as well as the person with dementia.

CHAPTER THREE

GETTING AN ACCURATE DIAGNOSIS

No two dementias are the same. Every person is unique and will present different symptoms. The first step toward an accurate diagnosis is to rule out anything that may mimic any form of dementia, such as a medical, pharmaceutical, or environmental condition that can cause memory loss. Many doctors, because of time constraints or their lack of knowledge, automatically assume that memory loss is a normal part of aging or, on the other extreme, believe that any memory loss is due to Alzheimer's disease. Many of my clients see me after they received a diagnosis of dementia from their primary care doctor or a psychiatrist. They are now seeking a second or third opinion. Some will walk away with a different diagnosis; dementia, the original diagnosis, was incorrect.

A misdiagnosis will affect the patient and the family both emotionally and financially. Every day, people are improperly diagnosed with dementia. A misdiagnosis will affect a person's ability to get not only long-term care insurance, which will help cover the cost of their care, but also other insurance that they may apply for in the future such as health, disability, and life. If you get your loved one diagnosed with memory loss before you have a good long-term care insurance policy in place and/or a good life insurance policy for them, then you are out of luck. If you think that your loved one is having problems with their memory, the most important thing you can do for them today is to get a good long-term care policy in place. Speak to several different insurance companies. Even if a person is no longer able to qualify for long-term care insurance, there might be other financial options that they may still qualify for such as a life insurance plan or annuity that you can later draw from to pay for their long-term care needs.

When a person is improperly diagnosed with dementia, it may affect the relationship that you have with them. Once the diagnosis is given, some caregivers pull back emotionally from their loved one because they believe that the person is going to forget them. Some caregivers prematurely take over responsibilities out of a belief that their loved one is no longer capable or feel that it's not safe for them to continue doing what they once did. Out of anger, some caregivers may lash out at their loved one. This anger is often due to frustration and grief they are feeling now that they've taken on the unexpected role of caregiver—they are grieving the loss of their imagined future. Some refuse to believe their loved one's diagnosis. Despite the brain scan and the obvious signs of memory loss, in order to hold onto normalcy, caregivers will continue to deny that their loved one is having a problem.

If you believe that a person you care about is having memory loss, after you have put in place a long-term care insurance plan, the next step is to find a qualified neurologist. Ask your doctor and your friends, and check the internet. In the short run, it may cost a little bit more out of pocket if the doctor is not in the person's health insurance network, or if the doctor is in another state. Because of the long-term effects of this disorder, my advice is no matter what the cost, you should find the best doctor you can. In the scheme of life, the cost of an accurate diagnosis is a small price to pay for you and your loved one's emotional and financial security.

Lesson One: *The Basics of HMOs*

We live in a highly specialized medical world. Technology advances daily in the medical realm and in research. A doctor who can keep up with all the changes and information on all of the new medication and techniques is an "überdoctor." Überdoctors are few and far between, but there are some out there.

The days of *Marcus Welby, M.D.* have come and gone, and so has the time when one doctor could treat you from cradle to grave. Up until the 1990s, doctors were more than just a medical expert; they also were trusted advisors, therapists, and a part of the family. I can remember from my childhood parties and events in my parents' home attended by doctors and their spouses; the doctors had at first treated us as patients and over time became close family friends. When I was growing up, doctors would make house calls, and even the family dentist would meet you at the office during off hours— and not charge you. Times—including the medical field and insurance—have changed. In today's world, just getting through to the receptionist can take hours, and then you may have to wait days, weeks, or months for an appointment. With the rapid advances of science and technology, a doctor needs to specialize in order to be financially successful.

Our relationship with our doctor is one of the most important ones we have, and yet we spend very little time with them. In the current system of insurance-driven care, your doctor has approximately fifteen minutes to spend time with you (and this number is on the high end). Here is the new medical reality: insurance companies will only pay the doctor for the first fifteen minutes (nine hundred seconds) they spend with you. Some insurance companies pay for even less time. Each additional second you spend with the doctor will affect the doctor's bottom line.

There was a time when I was not aware about how the health care industry worked. After graduate school and working for several years with doctors in a major hospital, I am now better informed and can share my knowledge with you. In order to understand the current system, you will need a short education as to why health care is where it is today.

Many primary care physicians are driven to reduce cost because of their contracts with HMOs (Health Maintenance Organizations) or PPOs (Paid Provider Organizations). These policies fall under the umbrella of managed care policies. Time equals money. Some plans reimburse doctors based on how few services they provide. The less money spent, the greater the doctor's reimbursement. Facilities such as hospitals and clinics are rewarded (reimbursed) if they discharge a patient prior to the allotted time. Translation: if they get you out of the hospital faster, they get paid more money.

The original purpose behind managed care was originally threefold. The first was to reduce medical costs. The second was to reduce medical errors. The third was that by assigning one doctor who is now your medical "gatekeeper," all of your doctors, procedures, and medications could be tracked, reducing duplication of services while improving the way your medical care and health care needs would be met. HMOs and PPOs were intended to put a stop to countless doctor visits, unnecessary surgeries, and the duplication of medication. The reality is that for many years, prior to the changes, the medical system was overused and often abused. There was a time when the medical system was a free-for-all. Doctors, hospitals, drug companies, pharmacists, and patients abused the system. At the first sign of a sneeze, cough, ache, or pain, a person would race to the doctor's office. And why not? The visit was paid for. Hospitals admitted and cared for individuals who stayed longer than necessary, and hospitals could charge the insurance company a ridiculously high markup for the medication and care they dispensed.

Because of skyrocketing costs in the health care industry, in the 1980s and 1990s some insurance companies came together and formed a coalition. They joined forces and came up with a plan that would lower their costs (payouts) to provide care and make a profit. The reality is that widespread abuse of the system is what caused this change. Today managed care plans, especially for the elderly, are the norm.

Often these plans look good on paper, but the choices within the plan can be limited. Let me explain why this is so. Once you sign up with a provider, you will need to choose a primary care doctor (PCD) from the plan's list. This doctor is now is in charge of when and if you can see another doctor, such as a specialist, and the medical tests that you can receive. At first glance it may seem that insurance plans have hundreds of doctors on their list to choose from. But after a person signs up for the plan, they may find out that the doctor they picked is no longer accepting new clients from this plan or is no longer on the plan.

Most plans will contract with a group of doctors that includes specialists. If a PCD directs a patient to a specialist on the plan, the PCD may get reimbursed by the insurance company. If a doctor refers a patient to another doctor who is outside of the plan, it will cost the insurance company more money. One of the most frustrating aspects of using an HMO is that in order for you to see a specialist, your PCD will have to write a referral. A referral to a doctor that is not on your plan may reduce the money that the PCD receives from the HMO. Some of my clients miss their appointment with a specialist because the required referral, which was promised by the doctor's office, was never sent. Often the referral wasn't sent because the cost may negatively affect the doctor's or HMO's bottom line. If a doctor sends out too many referrals, they may be dropped by the plan.

In order to make a living, many doctors will choose to sign up with several insurance companies. Today, almost all doctors have some form of a contract with a paid provider. Some insurance companies' plans pay a doctor whether they see you or not. Because of the low insurance reimbursement rate, many doctors have no choice but to sign up with many different insurance plans. This may be one of the reasons your doctor's waiting room is overflowing with patients and why your visit takes hours past your appointment time.

Doctors' contracts with HMOs and PPOs vary. Plans are specific in terms of the doctor and the medical tests or services they will pay for. If you choose to go out of your current plan to consult with a doctor, this may cost you more out of pocket, since some plans may not pay for a doctor who is not on their contract. But some insurance plans will pay for a visit when you seek a second or third opinion by a doctor who is not on their plan. Do not rely on the word of the insurance agent. You need to read the insurance plan carefully and understand what the plan will pay for. Ask a friend or family member to review the plan with you. Call the customer service representative, and above all, document everything (write down who you spoke with and what they said).

Even when you do all the right things, things don't always turn out the way you hope. My daughter needed to have her wisdom teeth pulled. I had never used my company dentist plan because I love my dentist, who is not on the plan. I asked my dentist about the cost of the procedure, and it was high, so I asked for a referral. That dentist's fee was lower, but still high. I called up the dental plan and asked them for a list of dentists on the plan that did extractions. They gave me a few, and I chose the dentist closest to my home. My daughter and I went for a consultation, and the procedure was approved by the insurance company. A month later my daughter had her teeth pulled, and on the way out I paid the co-pay. Eight months later a bill came in the mail telling me that I owed $1,500 because the insurance company denied the procedure. I'm still fighting it, even though I got a letter stating that they are sending me to collections unless I pay.

The reason that many people sign up with a managed care insurance company is that many HMOs advertise in the newspapers and on television and radio, or in some areas representatives will go door to door. The salesperson will tell a potential customer that all of their medical needs, including medication and all in- or outpatient services, will be completely covered under their plan. On paper, these plans look good and will often meet the needs of a healthy older person who does not have any form of dementia.

There are many insurance plans on the market, and choosing among them can be confusing. Costs and benefits will vary. Some companies put a cap on lifetime benefits. A million dollars may sound like a lot of money for health care, but in today's world, with all of the advancement in technology and new diagnostic procedures, this amount can be used up by one incident. Once you have been diagnosed with an illness or have had a medical procedure, unless you or your spouse is employed by a major company or corporation that includes provisions for you and your family, the insurance company will probably not insure you. If they do, it will cost a fortune. You may have a preexisting condition: age, for most companies, is a preexisting condition. The older we get, the more medical conditions the insurance companies believe will happen to you, and this may make you uninsurable or will require that you pay a higher premium. Previous medical conditions or surgeries may also make you uninsurable. If a company does insure you, they may exclude your preexisting condition for a year, for five years, or for life, and their plan may also contain a clause excluding any future medical conditions that might arise and/or be connected, although remotely, to your preexisting condition.

You should know that all personal medical information is shared among insurance companies. If a person has a history of alcohol or drug use, cosmetic surgeries, or cancer, if they are HIV-positive, or if they have any mental health condition such as depression, this information will affect their choice of health insurance policies and the probability of getting life or long-term care insurance.

One benefit some insurance companies offer is that all prescription drugs will be paid for. But many of these companies use a formulary, or a list of approved medications: the medication you use today may or may not be covered on the same plan next year. Who knows about the medication that is prescribed in the future? Some companies will pay for any medication a doctor prescribes, while other companies will only pay for a certain medication or a generic drug. Many health insurance plans may not cover new or experimental drugs. Under some HMO medication plans, if you want or need to use a specific medication that your doctor prescribes, the insurance company may require additional documentation from the doctor before it will pay. If a medication is not listed on the HMO's formulary, the HMO may require additional documentation that a certain medication is necessary and that the patient has already tried the generic version or another medication that didn't work well. Some doctor's offices may not have the staff or time to fill out these forms.

No matter which managed care plan you are signed up with, after one year you can switch to another plan. There is a specific time of the year where there is an insurance "window," and during this time you can change your current coverage without penalty. Find out in advance when this time is. Companies change, their benefits change, and—most importantly—your medical needs will change as you age. If you choose a plan based only on what is happening now, the doctor or medical plan may not be the best for your future medical needs. Before you automatically renew a plan- check the documents.

A note about private-pay practices: A growing number of doctors and therapists have chosen to have a private-pay (cash-only) practice. Because of the low reimbursement rate from insurance companies, and the endless paperwork that needs to be filled out and documented and when they factor in the months that it takes to get reimbursed (as well as the long wait for an appointment), many doctors have decided that it's not worth it for their medical practice to sign up for these plans. Many doctors and therapists now offer a private yearly contingency fee, as attorneys often do (called "consigner plans"), that will give you immediate access to the doctor or therapist to have your medical or psychological needs met.

Lesson Two: *A Brief Look at Medicare*

Here is a short Medicare primer:

1. Original Medicare provides basic coverage for hospitals (Part A) and doctors and outpatient services (Part B). It doesn't pay for vision, dental or hearing, routine checkups, or medication. You can go to any doctor or hospital that accepts Medicare. Medicare pays for

80 percent of the service. You are responsible for 20 percent of the cost.

2. Medigap supplementary insurance is a gap policy. This means that for a cost it will cover some out-of-pocket expenses not paid for by Medicare. Services will vary and will depend on the policy that you purchase.

3. The Medicare prescription drug plan covers only outpatient drugs and is intended for persons enrolled in Medicare who have no other drug coverage.

4. Medicare Advantage covers everything in the original Medicare but may offer lower costs and extra services. Check if the plan includes drug coverage. Once you enroll in an HMO (a managed care plan that requires you to go to the doctors in their plan), a PPO (a plan that allows you to see specialists without a referral and you will need to pay more to see a doctor that is out of the plan's network, a PFFS (a private fee-for-service plan that allows you to go to any doctor that accepts their terms), or SNPS (a special need plan for those in a long-term care facility that receives both Medicare and Medicaid). You will need to check each plan to ensure that Medicare will provide benefits.

You will need to choose the best plan for your loved one. In the reference section of this book you will find a list of organizations that can help you make an informed insurance decision. When it comes to insurance there are a few companies that I recommend for my clients. Keep in mind that any decision that you make is yours alone. You will need to choose what is best for you.

Lesson Three: *Navigating the Health Care System*

To get an accurate diagnosis of dementia, you will need to have certain medical tests and procedures done. Keep in mind that as a caregiver you are now an advocate. Persistence is important. To be successful, you will need to do your homework. When you choose to take your loved one to a specialist who is not on their current plan, the insurance company might not pay for some of the medical tests. Call the neurologist's office in advance, and ask the medical assistant or office staff what diagnostic tests your loved one may need to have after they have seen the specialist.

Neurologists use specific blood tests to rule out and diagnose dementia. For a good diagnosis, the doctor will need to review recent blood work and a brain scan. Ask the staff what type of brain scan they would likely order. Most doctors will want either a Magnetic Resonance Imaging (MRI) scan, which uses a magnetic field to create pictures of the brain, or a Positron Emission Tomography (PET) scan, which uses a tiny amount of radioactive material to produce pictures of the structure and functioning of the brain. If the person has a pacemaker, they will not be able to have an MRI, but they can have a PET scan or a Computed Tomography (CT) scan, which uses x-rays and computers to produce a series of two-dimensional images and/or a three-dimensional (3-D) representation of the brain.

This is not the time to be shy. Tell the doctor you are aware that there are medical conditions that can mimic dementia, and that it is in their patient's best interest to authorize the tests that can rule out any medical condition that is reversible. Keep in mind that with some insurance companies every test the doctor orders may have an effect on their financial bottom line. Make your request early in the month. This is the time when the doctor starts with a clean slate and may be more willing to send the patient for additional testing. Above all, remember that health care is a business. The long-term cost of caring for your loved one is also a business: your business. You are now the CEO of the company that is caring for your loved one, and you must take charge. Dementia is expensive, and as the head of your company you need to keep your costs in check, provide care, and do damage control.

If a person is having memory loss, it will be hard for any doctor to refuse to write a prescription for needed diagnostic procedures (they want to protect themselves from potential lawsuits). If the doctor stonewalls you (which they might because their bottom line is at stake), stay calm and in control of your emotions. Be assertive without being aggressive. In a soft and quiet voice tell the doctor, "I have been keeping detailed records of every conversation and have copies of all of the diagnostic reports." Calmly say that if it turns out that their patient—your loved one—has a condition, such as an undiagnosed brain tumor, or any other condition that could have or should have been ruled out early on, and might possibly be reversible, wouldn't they want to help? If the doctor refuses to run specific tests, ask them why they believe the test is not necessary. Your goal is to have the best diagnosis and treatment of your loved one. If you feel that you are being stonewalled, casually say that you are having dinner tonight with a family member or friend who just happens to be an attorney. Almost everybody knows somebody who is an attorney, and doctors do not want to be sued. Above all, no matter what happens, remain calm. Hysteria and theatrics will only go so far, and you will be labeled as difficult or an unbalanced caregiver.

If your loved one is not getting what they need from their current doctor, you may need to find a different doctor or specialist on their current health insurance plan or consider switching to a different insurance plan.

Almost everyone in the medical field uses contracts. Doctors contract with insurance companies. Insurance companies contract with the laboratories that do blood work, the pharmacies that provide medication, and even the facility that does brain scans. Keep in mind that depending on your loved one's current plan, and the one that their doctor is contracted with, the fewer diagnostic procedures that the doctor orders, the more it may add to their or the insurance company's bottom line. Be a smart CEO: get all the blood work and brain imaging such as a CT, MRI, or PET scan done in advance, with the person's primary care doctor. The same goes for any heart or brain monitoring. Bring all test results to the first appointment with the neurologist. This is especially important if you are paying out of pocket or traveling a far distance. The lab and test results you bring with you to the neurologist will ensure a quicker and more accurate diagnosis.

On a related note, one of my clients had an MRI that showed nothing remarkable. The neurologist ordered a PET scan, which showed a problem. I have read articles that recommend that you ask about the age of the machine that will be used. Some machines are old and no longer reliable. The insurance company will pay for the scan whether it's on a new machine or an older model. Moreover, all radiologists who read these scans are not created equal. Human error or an old machine can be the cause a wrong diagnosis.

There are some managed care policies that will be difficult to get around. Many of these are clinic-based. They may look good on paper and meet the current needs of a cognitively normal person who is either frail or elderly, but if you think that your loved one has dementia, you should consider reevaluating their current policy. If a person is sixty-five years old and a United States citizen and has paid taxes, they are entitled to a government program called Medicare. Depending on the person's current financial situation, they might qualify for Medicaid. If they have Medicare and Medicaid, they have now won the insurance lottery! There are many individuals who qualify for this government-paid plan and do not know it.

If your loved one has served in the armed forces, they are a veteran; you need to explore if they can qualify for additional health care benefits (if their spouse is a veteran, they may also qualify through their spouse's status). Some of the benefits they may be entitled to include reduced medical costs, free or low-cost prescriptions, and payments toward an assisted living facility or nursing home. They will not be reimbursed for past medical payments, but once signed up they will be entitled to future payments. Call the Veterans Administration, or check out their website. Some veterans' benefits are linked to specific years, days, military operations, or time served. You should also check out the benefits if the person was in the Peace Corps or another similar volunteer organization.

Veteran benefits will vary depending on where you live. Not every state will have the services that you may now need. When it comes to Medicaid, each state is different. Some of my clients have moved to another state to increase their benefits, and I also have clients who divorced (and still live together) in order to qualify for Medicaid benefits.

Using Medicare and Medicaid will open doors for your loved one. Although you will need time and a lot of patience, once you get through all the red tape and jump through all of the hoops, your hard work will pay off.

If your loved one qualifies for Medicaid, some drug companies will offer price discounts or provide the medication at no cost. If your loved one can't afford certain medications, they may be able to get financial assistance from some institutions that receive grants from the government or programs sponsored by drug companies. They will have to apply for these benefits, and they are not publicly advertised or well-known. Many people who qualify for these programs often slip through the cracks and do not receive the discounted or free medication because either the doctor's office does not have the time to do the paperwork, or they are not aware that there are funds available. As a loved one and now the CEO of their care, you will need to do additional research.

Lesson Four: Why Your Loved One Needs to See a Neurologist

Memory loss can happen at any age. Dementia does not just happen to people over sixty-five; it also happens to younger people in their thirties and forties. Dementia can occur for numerous reasons—family history, head trauma, or depression, to name a few. Any person who is experiencing changes in their memory should make an appointment with a neurologist. Not all doctors are created equal, and many doctors practice out of their field of expertise. Just because a person has the initials "MD" after their name does not mean that they are the best person to handle memory loss. If a primary care physician prescribes medication for memory loss without a full evaluation of the patient, they may be working out of their field of expertise. A neurologist will order current tests for blood work and brain imaging (CT, MRI, or PET scan), take a family history, perform a physical exam, and then, based on these results, make a possible or probable diagnosis. In the field of neurology, there are specialties. The doctor who read the patient's last brain scan may not be looking for dementia. To get an accurate diagnosis, you will need to find a neurologist whose specialty is dementia.

Over the last sixty years medicine and technology have changed and will continue to change. In today's world, being a doctor is a business—big business. Because of the money involved, many doctors choose to treat or feel they can treat every disorder. Many doctors will treat out of their areas of expertise. When it comes to dealing with dementia, this could be detrimental to your loved one's care. Since we are dealing with memory disorders, the most important doctor you should have on your team is a neurologist. If you have cancer, you see an oncologist. If you are having problems with urination, you see a urologist. If you are pregnant, you see an obstetrician. If you have a heart problem, you see a cardiologist. If you are having any type of memory problem, you need to see a neurologist.

You may wonder what a neurologist can do that your loved one's primary care doctor can't handle. Your PCD is not a specialist and may not be qualified to diagnose dementia in the nine hundred seconds that the insurance company will pay for. What the doctor often does is make a quick diagnosis. During their short time with the patient, they will make an assessment, give a diagnosis of Alzheimer's disease, and prescribe medication for memory loss.

I have met a lot of doctors who believe that memory loss in anyone over sixty is normal. Many doctors are not aware of or up-to-date on the medications that are available. Some doctors feel that the new medications are not effective. Primary doctors often miss the mark and prescribe medication for what they think is dementia when the person may actually be suffering from depression, grief, or a brain tumor. I am not saying that all primary doctors miss dementia, but as a caregiver you need to be aware that the trusted family doctor may not be the best person to diagnose dementia. So when should you seek out a neurologist who specializes in dementia? When you feel in your gut that things are not right or when the person you care for is put on medication but their behavior does not improve or their memory problems continue or increase.

Lesson Five: *How to Choose a Neurologist*

If your loved one has insurance through an HMO, they may have to choose a neurologist from their current plan. Many experienced neurologists work with HMOs or preferred care plans. So how do you and your loved one choose the person who is going to give an accurate diagnosis and will also guide you both along the way and support you through the diagnosis? When dealing with dementia, a good diagnosis is only the beginning. How the family or caregiver deals with the diagnosis is equally important. Since there is no cure or any medication that can reverse this disorder, you will need to find a center or a team of individuals that can help you. Ask your doctor whom they would send their loved one to. Ask friends what doctor they go to and why. Have family members look into the credentials of doctors and memory clinics. Check websites that grade doctors and the hospitals that they use. Keep in mind that no matter what plan your loved one is on, as a consumer they are entitled to a second opinion. I have clients who have paid out of pocket for third and fourth opinions. For them, it was money well spent.

All neurologists are not alike. Neurology is just one branch on the doctor tree, and they have their specialties too. Some specialize in Parkinson's disease, traumatic brain injuries, strokes, Lou Gehrig's disease (ALS), or memory disorders. A few neurologists are good and capable of handling many different types of brain disorders. Before you make an appointment with a neurologist, ask the front desk staff, "What is the doctor's specialty?" Ask how many patients the doctor has treated with the condition you are interested in. You are now doctor shopping. You want the best; don't settle for less. Also keep in mind that after you have met with the doctor, it is important that their personality fits with you and your loved one's needs. Some doctors are distant and may seem cold, while others may be more open and inviting. The doctor's style of interaction and personality are important. If you are a take-charge person, you may welcome a doctor who just gives you the facts. Some caregivers may need a doctor with a warm bedside manner who encourages and is open to their input and concerns. Remember, dementia can span twenty or more years. As a CEO, you are now building your dementia team.

Another important thing to consider is their office staff. A good diagnosis is one thing; how you and your loved one will cope with the diagnosis of dementia on a daily basis will depend on what support and resources you can access. Ask if the doctor's staff includes a person who has a master's degree in social work (MSW) or is a licensed clinical social worker (LCSW) experienced in geriatrics and dementia, or if they can refer you to someone who has these qualifications. In order to successfully deal with dementia, you will need to have on your team a person who understands and is trained in dementia to help you deal with your loved one's needs and the changes they will go through as the disease progresses. As a caregiver, you will need education, individual support to help deal with behavioral changes, and knowledge of available community resources. You will also need a person who can help you with the endless amounts of paperwork needed to qualify for many programs. This is where hiring an LCSW and/or a geriatric care manager will be invaluable.

A third consideration is location. As this disease progresses, and depending on a person's personality and behavior, it may become more difficult for them to tolerate a long car, bus, or plane ride. There may come a time when a person who has dementia may not feel comfortable or able to travel out of their neighborhood, or they may become so agitated that traveling is no longer an option. I have several clients who become violent, paranoid, or aggressive; have motion sickness; or are incontinent and unable to travel for short or long periods of time. In many of these situations, doctor's appointments will be missed. Missed appointments will affect the care of a person with dementia, including the management of their medication. If a person has not been seen by the doctor within a six- to nine-month period, the doctor's office may no longer be able to legally or ethically call the pharmacy for medication refills. In order to prescribe a medication the doctor needs to see the patient. Over time, some medications may no longer be useful, effective, or necessary. A person who has dementia will need to have their medications reviewed regularly and adjusted as needed.

Lesson Six: *What to Expect from the First Neurological Visit*

Your first neurological consultation for dementia will range from two to four hours. This may sound or feel like a ridiculously long time, but in actuality it is a short time for an accurate diagnosis, which is what you are looking for. This is going to be time-intensive for both you and your loved one. Unlike many other disorders or diseases that can be diagnosed through blood work or a body scan, there is no single blood test or scan that will easily diagnosis dementia. An accurate diagnosis will take longer than nine hundred seconds.

To get a good diagnosis your loved one (perhaps with your help) will need to fill out a questionnaire that is several pages long. It should include information about current and past medical history. They (and you) should be prepared to write in all the important data, including previous surgeries, vision and hearing problems, and current and past physical conditions. This form should also include family history, exposure to toxins, and personal life history such as trauma and physical, sexual, psychological, and emotional abuse. It should ask about recent changes in personality or behavior. Current and past medications should be listed. This is especially important if they have tried medication and suffered from side effects. Also, include any over-the-counter medicine as well as anything bought in a health food store, such as vitamins and supplements.

The reason behind this extensive form is to rule out possible factors that can mimic dementia. You or your loved one should feel free to write in additional information. If the person had hallucinations two years ago but no longer has them now, write it down. This is not the time to be embarrassed or think that a past behavior is no longer important. When you are dealing with a person who has any form of memory loss, these moments are important for a proper diagnosis. Past and present medication is important. Be sure to mark down what the person is currently taking and any medication in the past that was helpful or not effective. It's important to mention if your loved one has had hallucinations, delusions, or depression in the past and report any medication that has been prescribed or used to control current or past behaviors and medications that have caused additional problems. Also include a description of any recent losses in their life. The loss of a spouse or a family member or even a recent move from a familiar home should be noted.

Within this form there should be a two-part questionnaire that covers the person's current activities of daily living (ADLs), such as feeding, grooming, toileting, transferring, and dressing. (Remember that ADLs are those things that allow us to take physical care of ourselves.) The second part of this questionnaire should address the instrumental activities of daily living (IADLs), such as handling finances, remembering appointments, or being able to shop, cook, socialize, and travel, to name just a few. (Remember that IADLs are those things that allow us to live our lives independently in the community.) The scoring is divided into four parts: needs no help, needs some reminders, needs hands-on assistance, and is totally dependent on others. The higher the score, the more care or supervision a person needs. Recognizing what a person is capable or not capable of doing is an important part of the assessment because it helps determine what the person is able to do. Knowing a person's capabilities provides clues to potential problems. If Mom is having problems remembering appointments, she also might have problems remembering to take her medication. This is a tough form to fill out. Some people have never had to manage their finances or cook a meal. Many times caregivers have said to me or written on the form that the person has never done these things. I will point out that the question is not if the person has ever done these things. To fill out this form correctly, imagine if you were no longer available. Could the person do these things on their own, or be capable of realizing that they need help in this area and find someone who could help them?

The form should also include a depression scale. The Geriatric Depression Scale consists of 30 questions. This is an important form that should be filled out by the patient, not the caregiver. If need be, ask your loved one the questions, and fill in their responses. Many caregivers will fill out this form with answers reflecting how they think the person would answer this form or even simply their own perception of the situation. They answer based on what they see or believe or how they think they would feel if they were in their loved one's situation. Just because a person has dementia does not mean that they are depressed. A person with dementia may choose to stay home because it feels safer for them. They may stop previous activities because it is hard for them to get dressed. Some people, because of normal aging, may no longer be able to remember the rules of a card game, or because of medication they may now tire easily. Keep in mind that there are many reasons why a person may stop a once familiar and enjoyable activity.

Based on the answers you give to these questions, your loved one might be given unnecessary medication for depression. Caregivers often mistake their perception of a situation for another person's reality. As a caregiver you may miss the target. You filled out the form without asking Mom questions that are uncomfortable for you to ask or deal with. In this situation you are wrong: Mom is doing fine. Mom does not have depression or need medication. (On the other hand, you should consider that, as a caregiver, *you* might need counseling and/or medication to get you through this time. During the course of caring for another person, many caregivers will go through a period of depression.)

The next step for a good diagnosis is to have a professional review this form with you and explore additional information that the form does not cover. Frequently I will spend time talking with a family who has filled out the medical history form, and they will suddenly recall additional surgeries or medical problems. After reviewing the form, when I ask the client about their sleep habits, I am often told, "In order to get a good night's sleep, I take an over-the-counter medicine," which is not listed on the medication log. Through many years and after working with thousands of clients, I now refer to these forms as "meet and greet." I read what is written but realize there is more to the story. Through the form, I get a glimpse of the person and the family. The real work starts at the moment I ask questions that probe deeper than the yes-or-no answers on the questionnaire. I often joke that I am the warm-up act. After spending time with me and going over the forms, the family will start to open up. Family members may talk and argue in my office, but once they get into the doctor's office, all bets are off. When the family sees the doctor before encountering me, they have much less to say or overwhelm the doctor with information that isn't helpful. I fill in the blanks and give a heads-up to the doctor about what is happening and what to focus on.

The history you provide on the forms is just a starting point. During my interview with a caregiver or the family member, I will spend a lot of time going over the initial filled-out form and ask additional questions, probing further to find out more. This is when the actual diagnosis begins. Most of my clients come to our center for a second opinion. They were diagnosed by their primary care doctor with dementia or by another doctor. Many have been misdiagnosed. Over my years of working with people who have memory loss, I can count hundreds of people who have been misdiagnosed for dementia or behavioral problems and have been given or are taking medication they do not need.

My clients are amazing, and I learn from them daily. One of the clients I had in my office came to our center because of recent memory loss. Nothing in her past medical history pointed to any problem. I reviewed her depression scale, which, based on her answers, ruled out depression. I asked both the client and her daughter if there had been any changes in the family over the past year or two. They both said no. Forty minutes into our interview, after we had reviewed her form and I had asked many questions about her life trying to get to know her better, this strong, proud, widowed church woman broke into tears and told me in front of her daughter (who had filled out the forms) that three weeks earlier her son, who was sixty-two years old, had suddenly passed away. Fourteen years ago, after her husband died, this son had moved back into her house and provided strength and companionship. He also handled all of her financial needs as well as the shopping and the cooking. Her daughter was shocked: she had not realized the impact her brother's death had had on her mother, because "Mom has always been so strong." I recommended grief counseling, as well as family, church, and community resources. Her Mom was devastated and grieving; she didn't have dementia, even though her test scores were low enough to indicate dementia. Stress and grief can affect memory.

At her four-month follow-up appointment I had the opportunity to spend time with this client, who originally was diagnosed with moderate dementia; she was now clinically normal. I asked her and her daughter what had changed in their life. The daughter told me that she had followed my recommendations for individual and family counseling and enrolled her mom in activities in a senior center. Mom told me that based on our conversation and my recommendations she is now more secure, more independent and self-sufficient, and once again she is active in her community. She is continuing to deal with the grief of losing her spouse and her son. The bottom line is that she didn't have dementia.

Memory is a funny thing. Sometimes even the best of us forget things from our past, and we need someone to jog our memory. Sometimes it's not the actual question but the way the question is phrased. Once I asked a client if he was ever the victim of a violent crime—a standard question on my form. The client said no. I then went on to ask him several questions that are not on my form. I asked about previous head trauma. He said no. Something about the way he answered the question kept me delving further. I forged on: "You have never been in a car accident, fallen out of a tree, or gotten hit on the head as a child playing sports?" Once again, he said no. I was stumped; I sensed that something had happened, but I couldn't put my finger on it. So I kept going: "No falling out of buildings or boxing matches? Did you play football or soccer? A parachute didn't open?" He replied no to all, but in this last question I saw a spark of recognition in his eyes. As I was getting ready to go on to the next question, he looked at me and said, "You know, I had completely forgotten about it, but about fifteen years ago the plane I was piloting crashed. I was unconscious and in the ICU for four months." Memory is not always reliable or perfect.

To get a better understanding of each client, I will typically do two separate interviews: one with the client and another with the family members. Clients may lack insight into their current situation. A client may deny memory problems or think that their memory problem is typical of normal aging. Through the years, I have also learned that family members are not always the best or most reliable source. Some of the caregivers I see will either over- or under-report important changes. Caregivers have their own agenda. A caregiver may tell me that the person with dementia is able to do things that I know from their testing they no longer are able to do. Other caregivers will amplify psychiatric conditions so that additional medication will be prescribed to calm the person down because the caregiver needs to work, and if Mom is medicated, they will no longer have to worry about her. After interviewing the family, I am pretty good at figuring out who are the reliable witnesses and what the current situation is. I will pass on my insight to the doctor, but in the end, it will be up to the doctor to make the diagnosis.

The third step for a good diagnosis is a mental status assessment. The mental status assessment is often referred to as the Folstein or the Mini Mental Status Exam (MMSE), and it is a tool for the evaluation of dementia. This exam can help determine the severity of this disorder and can be used as a baseline to chart the course of a person's dementia. It is also a helpful tool to determine if the current prescribed medication is making a difference. The MMSE is composed of thirty questions that cover orientation, language, memory, comprehension, calculations, motor skills, visual spatial and auditory functions, and recall. The MMSE has been used universally to determine a person's current cognitive level. Recently another test was developed and is now being used: it is called the MOCA (Montreal Cognitive Assessment test), and some doctors are now using this to screen for mild memory loss. You should check it out on the internet. During testing, the neurologist and social worker will also be observing behavior, personality, level of alertness, cooperation, coordination, slowness of speech or thought, and the difficulty or ease a person has in responding to directions.

All new patients at our center are given the MMSE and, in addition, a more comprehensive neurocognitive evaluation that will include memory recall for short- and long-term memory, recognizing and naming of often-used and familiar items, comprehension (understanding what to do), praxis (hand movement), and simple math. I prefer to do the testing myself. For me, it is not just about the answers. I also consider how long it takes them to answer and the route they use to answer. I note, among other things, body movements, voice, and verbiage. It's not about how or when they got the right answer, but it is the time they took to correctly answer the question that gives me insight as to how well they are managing. They might give the right answers, but I clock their response time. Many people who have good cognitive reserve will be able to pass this test with flying colors. If they respond correctly but their response time is slow, my observance and insight will help with a good diagnosis and the future care plan. In the MMSE there is a math problem in which a person is asked to subtract seven from a hundred and keep doing this subtraction five times. When a psychologist administers the MMSE, if the person is not good in math, they will be asked to spell "world" backwards. The person will get credit for spelling the word correctly by a psychologist but not by some neurologists. Ask to see the exam, and look carefully at the results. I'm not good at math. If I were tested with the MMSE, let's just say I might be placed on medication.

The fourth step for a good diagnosis is for the doctor to perform a physical examination. Here the doctor is checking for physical changes such as stiffness, tremors, and problems with gait (walking and balance) and reflexes—for the physical signs of dementia. After the physical examination, the doctor will request blood work, which should include blood count, serum B-12, thyroid screening, a liver function test, basic electrolytes, glucose, and renal function tests. Because the brain will have changes with Alzheimer's disease, structural imaging such as a CT, MRI, or PET scan will be ordered. Brain imaging is used to rule out such things as hemorrhages, tumors, or a stroke. The imaging tests are invaluable diagnostic tools, but they also have some pitfalls. All brains are different. The scan may show there is a problem in the brain, but if there is no other scan to compare it with, the doctor may base the diagnosis on this scan alone. The patient could have suffered from brain trauma years ago, or maybe this is just how their brain is, and it could be something existing from birth. If possible, the person should get an MRI scan every few years, and then a neurologist can compare the scans. If the lesions are not growing or developing, then it might not be Alzheimer's disease. On the flip side, if there is damage to the brain, knowing the areas of the brain that are involved may help you understand the changes your loved one is now experiencing and help you as the caregiver deal with the changes.

By the end of the appointment, the doctor will make a potential diagnosis based on information from the medical history, family reports, social worker report, MMSE score, neurological test, and the physical examination. Some neurologists prefer to wait for the blood test results and brain images before they give a true diagnosis and prescribe medication. Some individuals, even without the diagnosis reports, will show clear signs of some form of dementia and be given medication before any test results come in. To postpone treatment of obvious memory loss until test results are available goes against the doctor's Hippocratic Oath. In the end, it comes down to a judgment call. If a person is having memory loss but the doctor is unsure of the cause, the doctor might not prescribe medication until they have received results of all the medical tests. Some neurologists may send a person for a complete neuropsychological evaluation, which is done by a psychologist to help with the diagnosis. A good neurologist will avoid prescribing medication unless there is a need. Many doctors will wait until they have all the results before they prescribe medication. You may feel that you are waiting a long time for the test results, but the goal is to have a good diagnosis.

Lesson Seven: *What to Bring to the First Neurological Visit*

As you now know, an accurate diagnosis takes time. The following list will help make the most of your time as well as prepare you and your loved one for the first visit:

1. One month before the appointment, call the neurologist's office and ask if a referral is needed. If it is, immediately call your loved one's doctor and either pick up the referral yourself or have the office fax the referral to the neurologist's office. I can't tell you how many times people have shown up for an appointment and the promised referral never arrived. Since many caregivers and clients come from out of town, this is a not-to-be-missed step. Make sure that you have verbal and/or physical confirmation that the referral has been received. To be on the safe side, have the doctor's office fax back to you the confirmation that the referral has been received.

2. When you call the neurologist's office to make the appointment, check that they are still on your loved one's current health insurance plan. Appointments are often made months in advance; the person you are caring for might have switched plans or may have been "slammed" (a company switched them without their knowledge), or the doctor's office is no longer accepting patients with their current plan. If the neurologist is no longer on their current plan and they still want to see this doctor, ask how much the visit will cost. All costs, including those of the office visit and tests, are negotiable.

3. Call the primary doctor's office, and ask them to fax over any blood work results. If the person you are caring for has a CT, MRI, or PET scan result in their file, make sure that the scan is sent to the neurologist. Call the neurologist's office to be sure that they have received the information. You should keep a copy for yourself, to be on the safe side. I also advise, if possible, to go in person and get the films or CD of the original test for the neurologist to review. Remember, the neurologist is reading the results from another doctor. It's better for the doctor to see and review the scan for themselves.

4. When you call the neurologist's office to make the appointment, ask if there is any paperwork that needs to be filled out. Trust me, neurology-related forms are long, taking anywhere from two to three hours to complete. There might also be questions you or your loved one is not sure how to answer. It is better to fill out the forms in your own home and be able to call other family members for their input rather than complete this form while sitting in an office with your loved one if they are anxious or hostile.

5. Arrive for the appointment prepared. Bring all of the patient's documents, such as their Social Security card, Medicare or Medicaid (if eligible) card, insurance information, and personal identification such as a driver's license, passport, or state identification.

6. Bring a sweater and some snacks. An office visit can take a very long time. It feels even longer if you are hungry or cold. Plan on bringing more food if the person has diabetes or low blood sugar. Dress in layers

for comfort. Bring a book or magazine that the person will enjoy reading or looking at.

7. If the person is incontinent, bring diapers, wipes, gloves, and a change of clothes. Many offices do not keep incontinence supplies on hand.

8. If the person wears hearing aids, make sure that the batteries are working and the devices are in place. If the person wears eye glasses, bring them.

9. If the person has a wheelchair and you are driving to the appointment, put the wheelchair in the trunk. Until you get to the facility you will not know how far it is from the parking lot to the actual office. Some medical complexes have very long hallways, and walking for some people is exhausting.

10. Bring all medication that the person is currently taking. It is also advisable to call up each doctor the person sees and have them fax to you their current medication log. This will be useful to check to see if the medication prescribed by their various doctors is duplicated (sometimes under a different name) or contradicts each other. Also, some elderly people have sleeping problems, and it is helpful to know if they are overmedicating themselves. Bring a list of all over-the-counter (OTC) medications as well as any herbal remedies and supplements that they are using (or have used). Before the office visit, go through the person's medicine cabinet, pantry, drawers, and refrigerator to check for any OTC medications, herbal remedies, vitamins, or tea. Vitamin E is a blood thinner; so are garlic and aspirin. If the person is taking a prescription

blood thinner along with aspirin, for example, this could be causing a medical problem.

11. Make a list of all your concerns. It is human nature to "go blank" in a doctor's office. Many of my clients' caregivers will discreetly hand me a letter that goes into detail about behavior or personality concerns. This way, concerns are not spoken in front of the client. I find caregivers' personal insights and questions helpful during our interview.

12. If possible, bring a tape recorder. A doctor's visit can be overwhelming. Record what goes on in the doctor's office, and play it back later when you are relaxed. You will be amazed by what was actually said versus what you heard or what you think you heard. You will be surprised by what you missed.

13. Bring lots of patience and a sense of humor.

Lesson Eight: *Getting There Is Not Half the Fun*

Making an appointment is one small step on the road to a good diagnosis. The next step is getting your loved one to the doctor's office. For some people, going to a doctor's office is a normal activity, and they take it in stride. For others, the doctor's office is a place to be avoided at all costs. A person who has memory loss may know that they are having a problem and may actually look forward—although apprehensively—to the visit. Others may deny or not recognize that they have a problem and refuse to go. Some people may be suspicious. They may forget what they had for breakfast, but they will remember that you are taking them to a doctor to check their memory and at the last minute refuse to go. No one wants to hear that they are having memory problems. Below is a list of suggestions on how to help a person who doesn't want to go to a scheduled doctor's visit. When in doubt, call the social worker before you approach a person with memory problems to find a way to successfully get them to the doctor's office.

1. If the person is functioning normally and independently, have them pencil in the appointment in advance so that there will be no conflict that day.

2. If the person is anxious, try not to give too much advance notice. I have found it helpful to just call them up and say lightheartedly, "Mom, I just checked my appointment book, and I totally forgot that you have a doctor's appointment tomorrow. I'll pick you up at [time], and we will go for lunch/dinner afterwards," or "Mom, Dr. So-and-so's office just called me to remind us of your appointment tomorrow. I'll pick you up at [time], and we will go to lunch/dinner afterwards." If you are living with the person and they are anxious, the best approach is to have a family member or friend call you a few hours before the appointment. Speak on the phone for a moment, and then casually turn toward your loved one and tell them that the doctor's office just called to confirm today's appointment. Put a smile on your face and say, "The doctor's office just called. Let's get ready to go, and afterwards we will go to lunch/dinner."

3. If the person starts to question or gets suspicious or anxious about going to the doctor, remain calm. Remind them that their favorite doctor made the appointment for them at the time of their last visit.

4. Do not use the term "Alzheimer's disease."

5. When you are pressed for more information, just say that all doctors now routinely schedule memory appointments for all of their patients over fifty-five (or the same year as the person's actual age), and assure them that the insurance company will pay for the visit. Say that this appointment is no different from a stress test, mammogram, or prostate exam—something they have every year.

6. If the person knows they are having memory problems and are scared of an Alzheimer's diagnosis, reassure them. Try saying, "Dad, I know that you are scared, and I don't blame you. There are many medical reasons for memory problems, and some are reversible if caught in time." Reassure the person by saying, "I'm here for you. We'll go together." Or say, "Dad, there are medicines available that can slow down memory loss. Let's see if they will help you."

7. Diagnosis day is not the day to drop Mom off at the doctor's office and come back later. Reassure her that you will be there with her at all times. If Mom says it's not necessary for you to go with her, don't argue. Agree with her, drop her off at the front door, park the car, and then join her in the waiting room.

8. People with memory problems may forget that they have a doctor's appointment. Call them in the morning to remind them.

9. If the person refuses to go to the appointment and says, "There is no reason to go. This is hogwash—I don't have a memory problem," or blames the problem on their spouse, calmly say, "Dad, I agree with you, and this way we can show Mom that there is nothing

wrong the next time she complains about your forgetfulness." You can also say, "Dad, Dr. So-and-so made this appointment for you. You don't want to disappoint him."

10. I advise some families to pick up the person from their home and just take them to their appointment. Sometimes being matter-of-fact works wonders. "Mom, I know that you do not want to go, but I'm picking you up at [time]." Make sure that you get to their house at least an hour and a half *before* the appointment to make sure that they are dressed, have eaten breakfast, and taken their medications. In some families, threats work well. "Dad, if you do not go to this appointment, I am no longer coming over to help with the grocery shopping/errands/lunch or bringing the grandchildren to visit." Use whatever works.

11. Sometimes you will need to use loving deceptions. In this case, I advise my caregiver clients to tell their loved ones that the appointment is for the caregiver, but that they want their loved one to come with them. "Mom, I have an appointment with Dr. So-and-so tomorrow at [time]. I want you to come with me—you know how nervous I get in the doctor's office."

12. It might work to tell Dad that you have to drop some papers off at Dr. So-and-so's office, which should take five minutes, and then the two of you will go out for lunch (or the drop-off is after lunch). Have Dad come in to the office with you. When you go to the front desk (call in advance so that the receptionist or the social worker knows of your plan), the receptionist says, "I know that your dad's appointment isn't for

three more weeks, but we just had a cancellation. Since you are already here, why not come in now?"

13. Schedule the appointment at the best time for your loved one. You want a good diagnosis. If Dad is not a morning person or is difficult to get up in the morning, he may not perform at his best during a morning appointment, and the diagnosis may not be accurate. Because the sleep-wake cycle varies for each person, schedule the doctor's appointment for a time that will be best for your loved one—not a time that is the most convenient or easiest for you or the doctor's office.

From my over twenty-five years of personal experience as a caregiver and as a professional who specializes in dementia, I have learned that to get a person who has memory loss into a doctor's office when they don't want to go will require creativity and perseverance. The suggestions above have worked for other people, and they may also work for you. Each person is different. In some situations I have found that using guilt or bribes (although this tactic may be uncomfortable for you) may be the only way to get a person who is paranoid or insecure into the doctor's office. As a caregiver, you are not being unreasonable or manipulative. You need your loved one to go to this doctor's appointment to get an accurate diagnosis so that you can plan for their future and yours. You will need to do whatever it takes to get them to this appointment.

Every day I get calls from anxious family members asking me for suggestions for getting their loved one to an appointment. Many caregivers jump the gun and tell the person that they have a memory doctor's appointment. Keep in mind that a person who has memory loss may be scared and paranoid. They are now hyper vigilant. For a person with memory loss, seeing a doctor who will check and confirm their memory loss translates to the idea that they're losing their minds and will spend the rest of their days in an institution. In this case say nothing about the doctor you are going to. Call their office social worker for suggestions and advice that is tailored to your loved one. Keep in mind that the goal for all concerned is a good diagnosis.

Lesson Nine: *A Few Final Notes*

1. Today is not the day to dress up your loved one. A lot can be learned from the way a person dresses themselves. If they normally dress themselves or if they typically live in one outfit, let them come as they are. Their current appearance will help with an accurate diagnosis.

2. Check off everything in Lesson Seven so that you will be prepared and calm. Your calmness will be contagious to your loved one.

3. Some doctor's appointments will take longer than others. No matter what the doctors front desk tells you, plan to spend an entire day.

4. Alert the staff immediately if a behavior problem happens in the waiting room. The office staff should be trained to deal with this situation and, if necessary, will bring you into an available office immediately.

5. Do not be afraid to complain if the wait is long. The squeaky wheel gets the grease. If all else fails, you can always leave. There is no reason after seeing any of the medical staff that you should wait for hours with a

person who has memory problems. No matter what the doctor's reputation, sitting in the waiting room with a person who is anxious or agitated for over one hour is unacceptable. Speak to the office staff. Some days there may be a medical emergency, and all of the clients will be put on hold. Emergencies happen, and this could be the day. If after a few appointments with this doctor you notice they are always running late, consider finding another doctor. Sitting in a waiting room with an anxious person who has memory loss will increase their stress and yours. This is not a good situation for either of you. If you schedule other appointments or plan another outing around this appointment, and the doctor is running late, you will be stressed. Stress is contagious. Once you feel stressed, so will your loved one. Down the road, stress may accelerate dementia. No one needs added stress, and no doctor is worth waiting hours for.

CHAPTER FOUR

MEDICATION

Once a diagnosis is given, the first concern for family or friends is, "Where do we go from here"? For most people, medication is their first thought. Caregivers want a medication that will stop the progression of memory loss, reverse it, or end a difficult behavior. What everyone wants is a pill that will return life to "normal," or to what it once was. As of today, there is no magic pill. A medication treatment approach will vary for each individual. The specific dementia disorder, as well as the stage the person is in, will determine the type of medication given. For individuals who have dementia and are now experiencing some troublesome behaviors, certain medications may be helpful, but for some people medication may increase the problem behavior.

Treatment of dementia can be divided into three categories: pharmacology, medical/surgical, and behavioral. I am going to discuss medication first because for many caregivers this is often their first line of defense against this disorder. Just knowing that there are medications that can control an unwanted behavior gives many people peace of mind. Medication has its time and place. The same medication that gives you relief may also have some pitfalls, including serious side effects. After an accurate diagnosis, the second reason that most people come to our center is for medication control.

Lesson One: *The Limits of Medication*

Today we believe that for any medical problem we have, there is a medication we can take to solve it. For many disorders that were once considered fatal, this is true; unfortunately when it comes to dementia, there is no cure. Despite what we have wished for, read on the internet, or heard from doctors or well-meaning friends, there is no magic pill that will reverse or stop the progression of dementia. There is no pill that will return life to normal or reverse the deterioration to the brain caused by this disorder. Many studies and scientific "breakthroughs" are helpful when it comes to understanding the causes of dementia and in directing science on the road to exploring and designing the future medications that may stop or reverse this disorder. For a person who is caring for a person with memory loss, the current research gives hope. But as a caregiver you still have to deal with what is known today. And as of today, there is no medication that can reverse or stop the progression of dementia.

There are only four medications that may slow down the progression of this disease. Depending on the stage and type of dementia, there may be some medications that may be helpful at some point to reduce your time as a caregiver and allow the person with dementia to remain independent longer. I say "may" because to date there has been no conclusive, unbiased scientific study that shows the effectiveness of any memory medications. Almost all of the clinical drug trials are performed or sponsored by the pharmaceutical companies themselves. (If you search the internet for "dementia," you'll notice that almost every website is sponsored by a drug company.) According to the *Wall Street Journal* and the *New York Times*, many of the findings from clinical drug trials failed to mention that the doctors who ran these studies have financial ties to pharmaceutical companies. Numerous reports have stated that many of the drug trial results are not accurate. Billions of dollars are spent and are earned worldwide from these medications. This is why I say that the medication *may* help a person with dementia.

Some countries outside of the United States are now questioning memory medications' effectiveness versus the cost factor. The concern is that the medications have a nominal effect—not enough to justify the current cost or to justify the side effects that many people report. European countries want to stop paying for these drugs because their independent studies have shown that the cost of these drugs in the private and public sector are not cost effective in the short or long term. When it comes to dementia, Europe is five steps ahead of the United States.

Lesson Two: *Understanding the Drug Companies*

Drugs are big business. Actually, drugs are a multibillion-dollar business. If you doubt this fact, just check the financial pages in any newspaper. Pharmaceutical companies are major players on the stock market. These companies spend millions of dollars each year advertising their drugs on television, radio, magazines, and newspapers. At the same time, drug companies give millions of dollars to doctors and their offices for promoting their products. They have done "data mining," where they use prescriptions to identify which doctors are prescribing their drugs and which doctors are prescribing the competition. Up until recently (before new regulations were put in place), the drug companies gave their sales representatives expense accounts that allowed them to spend thousands of dollars (depending on the territory) to wine and dine doctors and their office staff. Pharmaceutical companies often sponsored and underwrote all of the doctors' meals, rooms, travel expenses, and honoraria (payments to doctors for speaking and presenting) related to seminars and conferences. Without their financial help, many of the clinical studies might never have taken place. Medication is business, and for any business, the bottom line is profit.

It costs the drug companies from $500 million to over $1 billion to develop and bring to market the drugs that can help cure, stop, or slow down the progression of diseases. A drug does not appear on the market overnight. Teams of scientists, doctors, and technicians spend years working on a potential drug. Once developed, the drug needs to be tested. This is where clinical trials come in. In the initial phase, a small sample of the population is recruited to test the effectiveness of the drug. In this initial study (phase 1), one group of individuals are given the actual drug, while the other group receives a placebo (sugar pill). Some companies test the drug to learn about risks and side effects. If the drug shows promise, and the side effects are small, the drug moves into phase 2 of the trial. In the second stage, a larger test group where hundreds of people are recruited. Once again one group is given the actual drug, and the other group is given a placebo. Side effects and effectiveness are recorded. If all goes well, the drug moves into phase 3; this includes a larger group of people—hundreds or thousands of people—who are recruited and studied. Even after millions of dollars have been spent, many drugs never make it to the Federal Drug Administration (FDA) approval committee. And just because a drug made it through the FDA does not make it safe. Medications that have been passed by the FDA that have spent years on the market, and have been prescribed by many doctors are now being recalled because of serious side effects.

Over the past several years a few new dementia-related drugs under study seemed promising, but after phase 1 or in the middle of phase 2, the seriousness of the side effects put a stop to the ongoing trials. A few years ago, a vaccine was being developed that would not only stop dementia but reverse the changes in the brain that had occurred (it worked well in the laboratory with mice). Because of the initial success of phase 1 with humans, the study moved onto phase 2, when additional individuals were recruited. During the recruitment period, some individuals from phase 1 developed a swelling of the brain that caused a serious side effect: death. Even though this vaccine worked for some people and showed promise for others, the phase 2 trial was immediately stopped because of the percentage of people in the initial study who died. Scientists, doctors, and researchers are working at revising the vaccine and trying to pinpoint what caused this negative reaction in some people and not in others. There are currently a few new drug trials that seem hopeful. Even if they are successful, it will be years before these drugs are available in the United States.

Drug trials are expensive. Most studies are double-blind studies. This means that no one knows who is getting or not getting the trial medication. Neither the researchers nor the test subjects know who is receiving the medication or a placebo. In some studies the researchers know who is getting what. Many of these studies are done simultaneously at facilities around the world. This costs money. The medical facilities conducting these studies are compensated or granted money by the drug companies. Once a drug passes successfully through phase 3, then it can proceed through the process of FDA approval. It doesn't matter how successful a drug has been in Europe or any place else in the world; in order for any drug to be legally sold in the United States, it has to be approved by the FDA.

Namenda (Memantine) was used successfully in Europe for well over ten years, but it took an additional two years for the FDA to allow this drug into the United States. This means that for twelve years a medication that could possibly alleviate or help to slow down the effects of dementia was not available to many people who needed it in the United States. Even now, Europe is far more advanced in their treatment of dementia, both in their innovation of drugs and in their behavioral treatments.

Lesson Three: *Know Your Insurance*

Since the United States does not have a universal health care plan like Europe and Canada, we continue to rely on private insurance. People sixty-five or older who are on traditional Medicare can sign up for Medicare prescription drug plans. Some people choose to transfer their Medicare benefits into an HMO, which will pay for doctor visits and medication. Because of the changes in Medicare Part D, the plan they choose will determine the medicine their doctor will be able to prescribe for them. Doctors now have to justify why they want to prescribe one medication over another. Some insurance plans require that patients start with the older, less expensive medication and then show that the medication doesn't work before they will pay for a newer, more expensive medication. Some plans will not pay for Namenda until a patient has been on a cholinesterase inhibitor (such as Aricept, Exelon, or Reminyl—now called Razadyne) for at least three months.

In order to reduce medicine costs, many people in the United States are turning to our northern neighbor, Canada, to fill their prescriptions. Drug companies sell the same medication to other countries that they sell in the United States. As of this writing, any medication you purchase outside of the United States will not be counted toward filling the Medicare Plan D "doughnut hole"—the price that you will have to pay out of pocket or the gap in coverage that usually starts when costs exceed $2,700. Recently, some people who had been buying their drugs from across the border received letters from the Department of Homeland Security (DHS) instead of receiving the medication they had ordered and paid for. For a period of time, DHS confiscated medication that crossed the border. As of October 2006, DHS has ceased this practice. Buying drugs from Canada or outside of the United States can save money, but technically it's still illegal.

Many companies sell medication over the internet. How to tell the good from the bad is not so easy. You may have to spend a lot of hours on the internet finding a reputable company. You should know that to order medication on the web you will need a valid prescription. It will also save you money to buy a three-month prescription instead of a one-month prescription. Do not be tempted to save any additional money by buying anything more than three months' worth at a time because if the medicine is not effective or if the person is hospitalized, their prescription might be changed. Also know that in different countries, the same drug may look different. Some countries have a generic version of the drug that is not currently available in the United States. Some generic drugs for memory loss are now available in this country.

Recently I have read articles about counterfeit medications that are being made and distributed through the normal drug pipelines. Some of these drugs have ended up in the United States. Counterfeit drugs can be a problem no matter where you live.

As a caregiver, you are a part of the drug equation too. We all see the advertisements for new medication, and our gut reaction is to either pick up the phone and call the doctor immediately or ask about it during an office visit. The reality is that not all medications will work for everyone or should be used by everybody. Every medication will have some side effects, and if a person has additional medical problems, certain medications might not be appropriate for them. Before you pick up the phone to ask your doctor to prescribe a medication that you've seen advertised, keep in mind that there is no magic bullet or miracle drug that is going to return your loved one who has dementia to the person they were before. On the other hand, the right combination of medications can be helpful.

As a caregiver, you need to ask about the purpose of the medication, what you can expect, how long the medication will take to be effective, and the possible side effects. Just because a drug is prescribed by a doctor doesn't mean that it will be the best drug for the person you are caring for. As a caregiver you need to be proactive, take charge, and do some research. Some of the drugs that are currently being used to stop the behavioral disturbances in a person with dementia were never intended for this population. These medications were not tested on the elderly, whose bodies are different from a younger person and who are often on several different medications for other medical conditions.

The bottom line is that as a caregiver, you are the person who will ultimately choose what is best. Be a smart CEO: it might not be in your best interest or in the best interest of the person you are now caring for to passively accept what a doctor recommends. With the information I have given you, you are equipped to ask important questions. This is not the time to be meek. We are talking about your loved one and not a research subject. If you feel that your loved one is not getting the best medication or care, it will be up to you to confront the doctor. If the doctor is cold, arrogant, or dismissive when you ask about medication, find another doctor. Your loved one is not replaceable—your doctor is.

Lesson Three: *Current Medication*

The dementia-related medications on the market today may slow down the disease process in some people. Keep in mind that this disease is going to be unique to your loved one based on genetics, environment, current physiology, and age. These four factors will determine how well the prescribed medications will be tolerated and how well they may work. Despite what you may think or have heard, not one of these "memory" drugs is better than another. Some companies may spend more on advertising than others. Some doctors may be more comfortable prescribing a certain medication. Some doctors may be compensated for prescribing a specific drug. Depending on the person, a certain drug may be prescribed because it will be better tolerated or the dosage may be more convenient to give.

Medication may delay some of the symptoms of dementia, and this may allow the person to maintain their independence longer. This is especially important when it comes to their activities of daily living (ADLs), such as bathing, grooming, feeding, transferring, and toileting. For the caregiver, this means that the hands-on physical care you will need to do may be delayed. These medications may also help a person with dementia function independently in society for a longer period before they need additional assistance. But remember: medication will not return the person to their previous functioning. If a person is forgetful in turning off the stove or balancing the checkbook, they will still have forgetful moments even though they are on medication. Do not assume that because they are on a memory drug you can let down your guard. Dementia is a progressive and irreversible brain disorder. Memory drugs may help in some areas of a person's functioning, but not in all instances.

As this disease progresses over time, a person who has dementia will lose their ability to be successful and to remain independent in their independent activities of daily living (IADLs). They will eventually require some assistance and then, over time, become totally dependent on you or others for such things as grocery shopping, remembering doctor's appointments, paying bills, cooking meals, and getting around. When it comes to these daily activities, some people believe that if they see a decline in the person's abilities, the medications are not working, and they want to discontinue the medication. Know that IADLs are the very things that a person with memory loss will lose first. Often, once a person is no longer able to care for themselves, family members want to stop the medication because of the cost. Paying for expensive medication out of your pocket is a financial concern. For some families, the time that it takes to visit their loved ones or arrange for someone to come once or twice a day to give the medications is a financial and emotional hardship.

Let's face it: not everyone takes their medication with a smile on their face. If you are dealing with a person who is paranoid or delusional, you may have to use the Jaws of Life to get them to take medicine. I am not going to tell you to stop the medication if it is too expensive or difficult to get someone to take their medication. What I will tell you is that you have to be realistic. I don't know about you, but I would rather take over paying Mom's bills and buying her groceries once or twice a week than change her diapers several times a day. The purpose of the medication is to slow down the progression of the dementia. Keep in mind that each person's timeline through this disorder will be different.

For the treatment of memory loss, there are four medications that have been approved for dementia care: Aricept, Exelon, Razadyne, and Namenda. If your loved one has been diagnosed with dementia, they may be prescribed at least one if not two of these medications. Many primary care doctors prescribe these medications when there is concern about memory loss. The first three are in a class called cholinesterase inhibitors, which are designed to enhance memory and help boost levels of a brain chemical called acetylcholine by influencing certain other chemicals in the brain. Acetylcholine is released by a brain cell to transmit messages to each other. A cholinesterase inhibitor slows the breakdown of acetylcholine. What this simply means is that as we age, levels of the chemicals in our brains decline, and these drugs may replace what we normally lose.

The fourth drug, Namenda, is a medication that counteracts abnormal brain activity caused by another chemical called glutamate. Glutamate appears to stimulate the release of acetylcholine and to strengthen the way that certain receptors on message-receiving nerve cells respond to it. What Namenda does is to preserve normal synaptic electrical activity while suppressing extra-synaptic electrical activity. Think of this as a light switch that you quickly and continually turn on and off. The bulb will burn out. This is what may happen to the synapse in the brain. In a nutshell, these drugs are meant to slow down the progression of dementia.

To fully understand these medications, it is important to ask the doctor to explain how these medications work and what you can expect from them. Keep in mind that if your doctor cannot explain how the medication works and doesn't include the side effects, then they shouldn't be prescribing the medicine. Many people who are prescribed a memory medication are sometimes taking other prescription drugs because of additional medical problems. Normal aging involves some medical intervention. As we grow older, we are more prone to illness. Some medications should not be prescribed or combined with current medication. You need to speak with your doctor about these issues. If your doctor minimizes your concerns or discounts them, you need to find another doctor. When it comes to caring for someone with dementia, in order to be successful you will need to build a team. A difficult doctor is not a team player.

Lesson Four: *Side Effects*

Every medication will have a side effect. Some you may recognize, and others are so subtle that they will go unnoticed. Medication is considered a strange substance to the body. The power of suggestion when it comes to medication is powerful. For the "memory" medications that I have mentioned, side effects include fatigue, incontinence, stomach upset, nausea, and diarrhea, to name just a few. Many people stop using their medication because of these side effects. Additional side effects may include nightmares (vivid dreams), night sweats, impotence, constipation, dizziness, reduced appetite and dry mouth —and the list goes on. Some people experience none of these symptoms or slight symptoms. Before you stop the medication, you should speak with your doctor and see if the dosage can be changed or if the time that the medication is given should be adjusted. Doctors should prescribe medication based on its effectiveness as well as the convenience for the person with dementia and for their family.

Remember that a person with dementia will need additional help in remembering to take their medication or physically taking their medication. Some medications can be given in a single dose. Some are given two times a day.

Some are in pill form; others are liquid. Exelon has developed a twenty-four-hour patch that bypasses gastric problems and is applied once a day. The stage that your loved one is in, their current living situation, and their medical conditions will affect the choice of medication. The time you are able to monitor the medication is important for the effective dosage. If you or someone else is only available once a day, and the medication prescribed is to be taken twice a day, this can be a problem. For medication to work, it has to be taken at specific times so that the effective dosage level will be reached.

Some people, because of medication side effects, may need to lower the dosage so that the medication can be tolerated. A lower dosage of medication may not be effective. As a caregiver, you will need to use common sense. If a medication cannot be tolerated at a dosage that has been shown to reduce the decline of memory, you should ask the doctor if the reduced dosage is going to be effective. In some cases, a little medication is better than nothing; in other cases, no medication is better than a small dose. It is a tough decision to make. I have known clients who, because of medication side effects, could not tolerate the doctor's recommended dosage, but their family members kept them on the medications even as the person's quality of life was reduced. These clients were physically miserable. Many well-meaning families, thinking that they are doing what is best for the person with dementia, are actually hurting them.

Medication side effects are real. If a person who is given the medication becomes lethargic or has stomach problems, you will have to reexamine your belief and ask yourself, "Is what this medication supposed to do worth the price that my loved one is paying by feeling ill?" If a medication can slow down the course of this disease, but your loved one spends all their time sleeping or in the bathroom, is it worth it? If a side effect is sleepiness, the person with dementia may be more prone to falls. The purpose of medication is to improve their quality of life, not to damage it. If the person is having any side effects that affect their quality of life, you should talk to their doctor about your concerns.

Dosage for memory medication will vary. Listed below are some guidelines. But before your loved one starts any medication, you should confirm the dosage with their doctor. As time goes on, new medications will be introduced, but for now, these are the current medications that are typically prescribed:

Aricept: The person takes 10 milligrams (mg) once a day with food (after breakfast or lunch, whichever meal is bigger). It is recommended that the patient start on 5 mg for three to four weeks and then increase to one 10 mg pill once a day.

Exelon patch: The person starts with a 4.6 mg patch each day for four weeks and then, if that is tolerated, increases to a 9.5 mg patch. The patch is placed on the upper back, on clean, dry, hairless skin. The application site should be rotated each day to reduce the possibility of irritation. The same exact spot should not be used within fourteen days.

Exelon capsules: The person takes 1.5 mg a day for one week with food (after breakfast or lunch, whichever meal is bigger) and then, if tolerated, increases to 1.5 mg twice a day with food for one week. The person gradually increases to 6 mg twice a day with food, if tolerated.

Razadyne: The person takes 8 mg a day for four weeks with food (after breakfast or lunch, whichever meal is bigger) and then increases to 16 mg a day with food for four weeks. If tolerated, the person increases to 24 mg a day with food.

Namenda: The person takes 5 mg once a day for a week. The next week the person increases to 5 mg twice a day. If tolerated the dosage increases to 10mg once a day, and 5 mg is added later in the evening. The goal is 10 mg twice a day (10 mg in the morning and 10 mg in the evening). Namenda has been studied in combination with a cholinesterase inhibitor (the three medications described above), and some doctors will add this to one of the drugs listed above as the disease progresses or symptoms worsen.

It has been reported that the Exelon patch has reduced side effects and an increase in the medication dosage. If a person is having difficulty swallowing pills or is having stomach problems, check with their doctor to see if the patch or the Aricept ODT (oral disintegrating tablet) would be a better choice. Be aware that some people can have an allergic reaction to a patch placed on their skin.

For any medication to be effective, it has to be taken at designated times. If a medication reads "three times a day," it does not mean that the person should take it at breakfast, lunch, and dinner. It means they should take the medication in eight-hour intervals. If a prescription states that the medication should be taken four times a day, it means that the patient will need to take the medication every six hours. "Once a day" means a dose is given at one designated time and not randomly given within a twenty-four hour period. In order for any medication to be effective, the person must keep to a schedule. Ask the doctor what to do if a dose is missed.

Side effects are a major reason that people discontinue medication. Before you stop any medication on your own, call the doctor's office, and speak with the nurse or doctor. Some medications will need to be reduced slowly in order to avoid unwanted side effects. After any doctor's appointment you may leave their office with a handful of prescriptions for new medications. My advice is to introduce one medication at a time—slowly. When it comes to medication, start low, and go slow. Many of the elderly are on multiple medications that they need to be on just to survive. They may be on blood thinners, drugs to lower their cholesterol, heart medication, diabetes, prostate problems, etc. Any new medication that you now introduce may cause an additional medical or behavioral side effect. You will need to monitor your loved one closely for any potential distress. I recommend that when a person with dementia starts any new medication, they have someone living with them to make sure they take it according to the prescription and to monitor the side effects.

Lesson Five: *Be Informed!*

1. Unless a person has been properly diagnosed, ask questions, and research the medication before it is used. Remember that the purpose behind a thorough diagnosis for dementia is to first rule out any disorder that is reversible and to rule out any disorders that can mimic dementia, such as delirium and depression. A person who is having memory problems should not take any medication that may be ineffective, mask the problem, or make the condition worse.

2. The doctor should have a thorough history of the patient. When this history is given, current medications the patient is taking must be addressed. Just because it is purchased over the counter in a drugstore or natural food store does *not* mean that the medication is harmless or safe to use. This includes vitamins, cough and cold medication, allergy relief, pain relievers, sleep aids, and natural or herbal supplements. If it comes in a bottle, tea bag, or pill package, no matter what it is, it should be considered medication. It is a drug, whether it is or isn't FDA-approved. Just for the record, many of the natural remedies you find

in health food stores are not regulated by the FDA. Sometimes memory loss can be caused by medications or supplements. Some of my clients who have been taking over-the-counter drugs for years to fall asleep are now having memory problems. Anything that includes diphenhydramine or a substance that starts with "benzo" in its ingredients is a memory no-no. The same goes for any medication that promotes sleep, such as over-the-counter medications that have "PM" after their names. Using these products may cause next-day drowsiness, constipation, or an increased heart rate in some people. Even common medications that have acetaminophen may cause liver failure in some people.

3. Buy a physician desk reference (PDR). It can be purchased in drugstores, from bookstores, or over the internet. Because the elderly take many different medications, you should know what the possible side effects are as well as the dosage and the times that the medication should be taken. I have many clients whose medication causes them problems, such as fatigue or incontinence. Combining medications that have the same side effects will increase these kinds of problems. Unfortunately, many doctors will prescribe another medication to combat a side effect, which not only adds an additional medication in the patient's daily schedule but may be unnecessary. Ask your doctor to review all the current medication, check for possible duplication of medicine, review the herbal supplements as well as over-the-counter drugs, and then determine whether the current medications should be increased, reduced, or discontinued. You can also ask your pharmacist to

review the medications. On my team I have a senior pharmacist who reviews my client's medications for possible drug interactions and side effects.

4. With any medication the rule of thumb is to start low and go slow. Medication may have some unwanted side effects. Before you leave any doctor's office with a handful of new prescriptions, ask the doctor in what order your loved one should start the medications. Medication affects each person differently. Some people may tolerate and process certain medications better than others or, when they are combined, may suffer from drug interaction side effects. Unless directed by the doctor, under no circumstances should the person with dementia begin taking all of the new medications at one time.

5. Before leaving the doctor's office, make sure that you review the dosage and times that the medications should be taken. Some medications may need to be taken on an empty stomach; others may need to be taken after a full meal. Review the current medications with the doctor, and ask about possible drug interactions. Adjust the medication schedule accordingly. If after taking the medication your loved one feels ill, it might be a side effect of the medication. I often suggest to clients that when they start to take any new medication, they keep their routine as simple as possible and keep a medication log. If they are planning a trip, they should postpone taking any new memory medication. The last thing that anyone needs to have is a side effect when miles away from home and far away from a familiar doctor.

6. Ask the doctor if there are any specific instructions for taking or avoiding certain foods with the medication. Some foods such as grapefruit or orange juice can increase or decrease the effectiveness of some medications. Ask about adding dietary supplements to replace nutrients that are no longer absorbed into the body because of the medication.

7. Remember to tell the doctor of the patient's current activities. Some medications include a warning to avoid heat. This includes hot showers, heated pools, saunas, or exercise during certain times of the day. The elderly are more vulnerable to climate changes; they feel the heat and cold more than younger people. Some medications can make a person more sun sensitive. Sun not only provides us with vitamin D but also helps us to set our internal body clock, which allows for sleep. If you expose someone to sunlight while they are on a medication that is known to cause sun sensitivity, be aware that they may sunburn more quickly. And remember, as we age, our skin becomes thinner; this can cause additional problems in the elderly.

8. Report any adverse changes or side effects to the doctor as soon as they occur. Some medications may make symptoms worse before they improve, and it's better to be safe than sorry. Because each person is different and their dementia is different, the side effect of a certain medication may have the opposite effect of what the medication was prescribed for. For example, an anti-anxiety medication that should calm a person could make them restless or nervous. I always inform my clients that if they have any problem or concern, they should call their doctor's office immediately.

If symptoms are severe, such as vomiting, nausea, disorientation, or delusions, and you cannot get in touch with the doctor's office because it is after hours, call 911. If the symptoms are severe, do not wait for a return call from your doctor—call 911. Even if you reach the doctor, at this point there may be nothing that they may be able to do over the phone. The doctor will tell you to call 911, and they will meet you at the emergency room. If the person is in distress, call 911 and then the doctor. I keep stressing the "call the doctor" point because many insurance companies require this step for reimbursement.

9. Be extremely careful if your loved one lives alone and is prescribed a new medication. Medications may have side effects such as fatigue, nausea, or dizziness, which can lead the person to inadvertently harm themselves. If they are tired, they are more prone to have accidents. Dizziness can lead to falls. Nausea will mean loss of appetite. With loss of appetite comes dehydration, which will increase memory loss and cause behavioral problems. Even when the medication is making them sick, many people will continue to take them. The problem is that if they are not eating or drinking liquids, and continue to take their prescribed medication, they may become sicker. If they are tired, they may lose their appetite and not eat; they may become forgetful and not turn off the stove or be more prone to falls. Taking medication without proper supervision is an accident waiting to happen.

10. Once again, before you discontinue any medication, speak to the doctor or to their office staff first. Some medications will need to be slowly reduced. With

other medications, the person may be able to stop using them without any side effects. The same rule applies to discontinuing medication as it does when starting them, but in reverse: stop slow; decrease low. This is especially important for any medication that has been taken over a period of time.

11. Be sure that the medication is taken. Do not rely on the word of your loved one that they have taken or are taking the medication. Many people with dementia assure their caregivers that they have taken the medication when they haven't. During your next visit, count the pills that are still left in the medication bottle. Do the math. Look at the date that the prescription started, and subtract from the current date. How many pills are left?

12. Depending on the stage of dementia, if a person is suffering from paranoia they will be wary about taking any medication and can be incredibly crafty about hiding pills. You see them take the medication and assume that they swallowed the medication—wrong. Many people hold the medication in their mouth until they have an opportunity to get rid of it. I found many of my mother's pills jammed into parts of her bedding. Clients who saw their loved ones take the medication have told me that they later found pills hidden in the bedding, spit into a napkin, or hidden in a drawer. You will need to make sure that the medication is actually swallowed.

13. It's not uncommon for a person to be taking over-the-counter medications that you might not be aware of. Check cabinets in the kitchen and bathroom and

their night stand for additional medications, vitamins, and alternative medicines that they might be taking and have forgotten about. Some of my clients are on blood thinners, aspirin, and vitamin E—not a good combination, especially if they need emergency surgery for a heart problem or an accident, such as a fall. I also have clients who take their spouses' medication. Many times one spouse is on a particular medicine and will then share it with their partner. Because it is not the client's prescribed medication, they will not add it to their current medication list.

14. Inform the doctor of any medication changes. Since people see their primary care doctors more often than specialists, they often change or add to the patient's medication based on information from the patient. Many of my clients have been switched from one memory medication to another because they told their doctor that they didn't feel their current medication was working. Many in the elderly population are too embarrassed to tell one doctor that they went to another doctor, and the medication changes go unchecked.

15. If possible, do not tell a person with memory problems about potential side effects. Many people with dementia suffer from paranoia, and they will remember the side effects and will use the side effects as an excuse to stop taking the medication. A paranoid person will not want to take any medication. Most of us are aware of the placebo effect. This is where you expect a medication to work, and so it does. There is also an effect that you should be aware of. It's referred to as the "nocebo effect." This is when expecting to

feel ill can bring on illness. Studies have shown that patients forewarned about possible side effects are more likely to have them. A person's expectation of a medication will have an effect. I have found that when I mention in front of the patient possible side effects, they will have a medication reaction and will discontinue the medication. I now advise the caregiver not to mention adverse side effects that may occur in order to reduce the nocebo effect.

16. Ask the doctor what to do about a missed dose. Some of my clients have paid caregivers for five days a week, and a family member comes in on a Saturday or Sunday. Because of a change in their schedule they may forget to take their medicine. You need to know what will happen if they miss a dose. Another situation is hospitalization. When a person is in the hospital, they may get a new doctor who changes the current medication and prescribes new medication. Speak to this doctor before you continue any previous medication that was given before hospitalization. Ask after a hospitalization how long they will be on the medications that are now prescribed. Once again, you will have to review the medication and ask the doctor about possible side effects. Any medication that was given prior to hospitalization will need to be reviewed and possibly discarded.

17. Sometimes a drug is not covered by the person's health insurance plan. Will they be able to pay out of pocket for this new drug? If paying for this new drug will mean that they have to cut back on necessities such as food or utilities, you need to speak with their doctor.

Ask if there is a generic or older medication that can be substituted.

18. A person with dementia, depending on their stage of this disease, can have certain behavioral problems. Behaviors come and go, but many people stay on a medication far longer than they should. Once the behavior has passed a three- or six-month point, you should ask if the medication is still needed or could be reduced.

19. Always ask for samples of any new medication. Most doctors receive sample packages from the pharmaceutical companies. There is no reason to go out and buy a month's supply of expensive medication only to find out that it doesn't work as intended or causes intolerable side effects.

20. Check the spoon. When giving medication, the dosage matters. Many of us throw out the dosage cap that comes with the medication when it gets gummed up. When my kids where little and needed antibiotics I bought a dosage spoon from the drug store and then lost it. I thought that I could gage the dosage by using one of my teaspoons. You need to know that the sizes of teaspoons or tablespoons are different for each silverware set. Years ago I noticed when I gave the one teaspoon of antibiotics to my daughter that should have lasted ten days, only made it through eight. She lived, but it was a wake- up call for me to buy a plastic dispenser spoon each time she was given a new liquid medication. Adults normally take pills, but there may come a time when they can no longer swallow pills. There are some medications that are in liquid form

such as cough and cold medication, constipation, and pain relief. Using a tea or tablespoon from your kitchen may be the cause of under or over medicating your loved one.

Lesson Six: *The Dangers of Self-Medication and Dementia*

Many of my clients self-medicate themselves. Some use alcohol, others use over-the- counter drugs, some use prescription drugs, and some use "natural" homeopathic medications. I also have clients who use "natural" herbs such as marijuana. People will use a medication that has been prescribed for another person because it is convenient or to reduce their medical costs. Many of the clients I see combine at least two of the above. Any combination like that can cause additional memory problems.

Alcohol use in the elderly is often unreported and discounted. I had an eighty-five-year-old client who said that she only drank two drinks per day. After scanning her original intake chart, I saw that she was still drinking. The patient said that once she took the sleep medication that was prescribed she had heart palpitations, so she stopped her medication. The daughter who attended this office visit told me (in front of her mother) that after one drink, her mother had no recollection of anything. As an addiction specialist, I know that unless a person has a specific gene or a history of incredibly low tolerance to alcohol (which does happen), a person who has one drink daily is not going to go over the edge—unless they are underreporting their drinking or possibly mixing alcohol and medication. I gained this client's trust and then slowly introduced the reality that alcohol and any medication is not a good mix. If I relied on the information from her initial interview, it would seem that this client had two glasses of wine, which would be approximately six to eight ounces a day. Once I got her comfortable, it turns out that her two drinks consisted of three ounces of vodka with a splash of cranberry juice. It turns out that she was drinking six ounces of vodka nightly and *then* taking her prescription medication to fall asleep. No wonder she had heart palpitations and memory problems!

This client is not unique. Many of my clients drink, and their children or spouses are not aware of the extent of their drinking, how it affects their loved one's memory, or the side effects that arise once they combine alcohol and medication. Many independent living facilities and assisted living facilities have a nightly or weekly happy hour. For a person with no memory loss, these events provide a welcome normalcy and socialization. But for someone with dementia, they are risking their health by combining alcohol and medication.

As a caregiver, you need to be alert to the possible interaction of medication and alcohol. Alcohol also affects nutrition; many people who drink either reduce their food or eat too much. You should also know that alcohol will affect sleep. It may put a person to sleep, but eventually they will awake in the middle of the night and have difficulty falling back to sleep. Alcohol also dehydrates the body, causing memory loss and behavioral problems. Alcohol may cause an unnecessary slip or fall and nutritional deficiencies such as vitamin B, which can escalate dementia.

Lesson Seven: *How to Tell If the Medication Is Working*

By now, I am going to sound like a broken record: as of today, there is no cure for dementia. The medications currently available can only slow down the disease process in some people. Medication cannot reverse this disease or stop the progression. Medication is only capable of doing so much. This may sound harsh, but there is no magic bullet. There is no medication that will return your life or the life of your loved one to what it was originally. You are dealing with a progressive irreversible brain disorder. Medication *may* be able to slow down the progression of this disease, but nobody can say that it will for certain.

One of the most frequently asked questions in my office is "Is this medication working?" There are some ways to tell clinically, but there are other factors that will need to be addressed before a change of medication should be made. In the previous chapter, I explained neurological testing. The Folstein, also known as the Mini Mental Status Exam (MMSE), is one of the tests used. This test can provide a baseline for your loved one's current mental state. Each time they come for a follow-up appointment, the same test will be repeated. By comparing past and present scores and doing a thorough psychosocial evaluation at each visit, the doctor will be able to determine if the medication is working.

You must keep in mind that memory medication is not magical. The sole purpose of memory medication is to slow down the progression of this disease. End of story. Period. Nothing more. The purpose behind these medications is to help a person maintain a current level of functioning. The Folstein test can show one level, but it is not the most important level. During the follow-up visits I will ask clients and caregivers how things are going at home. This is where my concern lies. No matter how well a person tests, if they are now having problems finding the bathroom, eating by themselves, bathing, grooming, or just getting around, then the medication should be reviewed. Realistic expectations must be taken into account. If the person is no longer able to do the taxes or balance the checkbook when they used to be able to, there is no medication that will return them to those skills. As dementia progresses, you will have to offer more assistance, and over time you will become totally responsible for past chores or tasks that the person you are now caring for one once did.

So how do you know if the medication is working? You know the person you now care for. As the dementia progresses, no matter what medication is given, you will need at some point to step in and provide additional assistance. If the person with dementia can tolerate the medication and continues to maintain their quality of life such as feeding themselves, dressing with assistance, going to the bathroom with some help from you, and taking a bath with either your verbal or your physical help, and if they are capable of being left home alone, then the medication is working. If a person is able to go out and socialize, attend functions or family gatherings, and can enjoy this time, then the medication is working. Remember, medication can only slow down this disorder. It cannot stop it. When the time comes that you need to do everything for another person, then the medication may no longer be necessary. I say "may" because people do not lose all of their functions at one time. Your loved one or the person you are now caring for may need additional assistance in some areas but still be capable of functioning with minimal help in other areas.

As a social worker, my main concern is how well the person is functioning and how well the caregiver is dealing with the changes. I want to help caregivers help themselves and, at the same time, understand and help the person with dementia. My job as a therapist is easy compared to yours as a caregiver. You live with this every day. How do I know and understand what you are going through? My mother who had dementia lived with me and my family for sixteen years. Years before we lived together my days revolved around her care from a distance. I have lived with her and her decline, and I have been powerless to stop it. My children and I have experienced the most difficult of behaviors. I have also seen firsthand the side effects and complications that medication can cause. Just like you, I have been on the other side of the phone listening to a voice message at her doctor's office and feeling hopeless because nobody is there. I know what it is like to wait by the phone all day for a return call from the doctor's office—which sometimes never comes.

Lesson Eight: *Medical and Surgical Interventions*

I am not a neurologist, but I am lucky enough to work with some of the best on the East Coast and have met some of the best on the West Coast. Through them I have learned that memory loss is not always dementia nor is all memory loss always Alzheimer's disease. In chapter 2, I mentioned some of the different forms of dementia and the medical conditions that can look like dementia but aren't dementia. Earlier I told you why your loved one with memory loss should see a neurologist who is a specialist in dementia. I am now going to focus on two of my most recent cases. Their names have been changed to protect their privacy.

Audrey was seventy years old, and her personality and memory had significant changed. She was repetitive, forgetful, and obsessed with writing her life story to pass down to her children. According to her family, over the past three years her memory continued to decline, and she became irritable, argumentative, and childlike. Her primary doctor and first neurologist gave her a diagnosis of dementia and put her on medication. Audrey continued to decline. When I first met with Audrey and her family, we discovered through the interview process that it appeared she had a form of dementia, but something didn't add up. In the neurological testing, Audrey scored in the mid-range for moderate dementia. I learn a lot from watching families and caregivers interact in our waiting room. Audrey was writing a book for her daughters on how to live life. She brought this book with her and continued to write while speaking with other clients in the waiting room coherently about the importance of motherhood.

Listening to Audrey, I realized that what she was saying made sense. Perfect sense. When I presented the case to the doctor with her scores, I also included my observations. Yes, she has memory loss, but she also had long rational moments and conversations on topics that are not typical of a person who had her diagnosed stage of dementia. Another MRI was ordered and read by our doctor. Audrey had a brain tumor in her frontal lobe that was affecting her behavior and causing her memory problems. She had surgery, and her recovery is ongoing. Her memory has improved, and her behavioral problems have stopped. Audrey still needs some help with her daily functions but much less care than before her surgery, and she is no longer having memory decline.

The next case is of a person who was also given a diagnosis of dementia. Bob was having memory loss, and his doctor put him on medication. Bob's son contacted our center after he noticed that the medication that the primary doctor gave him was not working. Instead of getting better (remember, the goal of medication is to stabilize and slow down the decline) his dad was no longer interested in things that he once enjoyed and, most importantly, was always tired. I used to joke, "This is not rocket science," until I met Bob. He worked for many years at NASA and was a rocket scientist. Bob's family brought him to our office because of his memory loss. I met with the family and tested Bob, and he did have memory problems. During the physical exam the neurologist ordered additional tests. Bob had normal pressure hydrocephalus (NPH). This is where the cerebrospinal fluid builds up, causing ventricles in the brain to enlarge and putting pressure on the nerves that affect memory loss, bladder control, and gait (walking). If not caught in time it can cause permanent brain damage. Bob had surgery in which a shunt was implanted to drain the excess fluid from his brain. Bob's memory has improved, and he recently moved back into his own home after living in an assisted living facility.

Audrey and Bob are not unique. Many individuals are misdiagnosed with dementia and actually have a reversible type of memory loss. I see a few cases like this each year. A good diagnosis and proper and timely medical or surgical intervention can help a person and their family member deal with a problem that can mimic dementia.

Lesson Nine: *Medication and Difficult Behaviors*

Unwanted behaviors are sometime called difficult behaviors; I call them challenging behaviors. People with dementia, because of their behavior, cause their caregivers to be challenged mentally, emotionally, and physically. The repetitive questions, the verbal accusations that you or someone else is stealing from them, the endless walking around (pacing) with no purpose, or seeing things that no one else does: over time, living in this environment will drive any normal person crazy! The most mundane thing can set a person with dementia off. In the next chapter, I will explain in further detail as to why these behaviors happen and how to deal with them. Many caregivers believe the only way to stop the behavior is with medication. So I will now discuss some popular medication interventions that address behavior problems.

Keep in mind that the current medications on the market and the ones most frequently prescribed were originally intended to be used by people who are years younger and physically healthier than your loved one may be. These drugs were also originally developed and intended to help people who have been diagnosed with schizophrenia, bipolar disorder (also known as manic depression), or clinical depression.

The most troublesome behaviors fall into five main categories: delusions, hallucinations, agitation, aggressiveness, and insomnia. People who have delusions are extremely suspicious. A delusion is a false belief. The most common delusions held by people with dementia are that their house is not their home, people are stealing from them, you are not who you say you are (spouse, child, friend, etc.), or people are watching them. They will say that people are breaking into their home, the people on television are watching them, their spouse is having an affair—the list of delusions is long. Some doctors will prescribe an antidepressant, thinking that some of the delusions are caused by depression. They may also prescribe an anticonvulsant or an antipsychotic medication. Be aware that the side effects of some of these medications may be cardiac problems, stiffness, tremors, and forgetfulness.

Hallucinations are sometimes harder for a caregiver to deal with than delusions. A person who has hallucinations will see or hear things that are invisible or inaudible but they believe are real. They will see something (people, animals, or insects) in the room or on their body. They may hear people talking, a doorbell ringing, or dogs barking. They may smell odors that no one else can. They may feel something crawling on their body. Hallucinations are real to the person who has them. People with hallucinations are more apt to act out or act on the hallucination. Younger people who have hallucinations are often diagnosed with schizophrenia. The typical treatment for this disorder is antipsychotic medication, which may cause additional functioning loss to their brain. Many people with dementia can vividly recall their hallucinations. Many of my clients will tell me what they see, and in the next sentence they will admit that what they saw wasn't real. None of the dementia patients I spoke with had hallucinations that caused them to want to harm themselves or others. Hallucinations happen frequently with people who have a form of dementia called Lewy Body disease. When a person has this form of dementia, some of the medications prescribed to stop a behavioral problem may cause additional behavioral problems.

Agitation can be a major source of irritation for the caregiver. When a person is agitated, they fidget. For hours on end they will engage in repetitive, nonproductive movements, such as opening and closing a purse, going through drawers, combing their hair, packing and unpacking, folding clothes, or picking at their skin, to name just a few. To calm these unwanted behaviors, doctors may prescribe a low dose of Trazodone, which is sometimes combined with an antidepressant, anticonvulsant, or antipsychotic.

Aggressiveness is by far the most difficult behavior to deal with. A person who is physically or verbally aggressive is a threat to themselves and others. A person who is aggressive is now in a primal fear mode. Their adrenaline is pumping, and they are in "fight or flight" mode. Many choose to fight. Physical aggression is dangerous to the caregiver. A person who is aggressive can succeed in hurting the caregiver. Antipsychotic drugs are often prescribed to calm this behavior.

The most frequent phone calls I receive are due to either the client's or the caregiver's lack of sleep. If the client is not sleeping and is bouncing off the walls all night, the caregiver will not be able to sleep. Lack of sleep will cause additional irritation, agitation, aggression, and memory loss. Lack of sleep will typically cause both the person with memory loss and their caregiver to have behavioral problems. A person who has dementia may reverse their sleep pattern and spend their day sleeping and then be wide awake at night. After night one, two, or three of not sleeping, the caregiver will pick up the phone and call the neurologist's office and hysterically report this current behavior. I've been there and done that. The office will prescribe a medication to calm a person and help them sleep. The problem stops, and often the quality of life of the person with dementia declines because they often stay on the medication long after the behavior has passed. Medication that calms a behavior and is used over a period of time is a form of restraint.

Medication that is prescribed for difficult behaviors may have additional side effects, and the person taking the medication should be closely monitored. These drugs may not have been tested on the elderly. Many of the drugs used for behavior problems are used "off label," which means that some doctors found that the drugs worked in ways that they were not initially approved or intended for.

Below is a list of commonly prescribed medications that are often used to treat behavioral problems for persons with memory disorders. You need to know that some of these medications may take between four and six weeks to work and that all drugs should be taken with caution. No medication should be taken unless prescribed by their doctor. I have listed both the pharmaceutical name and the generic names:

- Celexa (Citalopram) is used to reduce depression and anxiety.
- Depakote (Sodium valproate) is used to treat severe aggression.
- Remeron (Mirtazepine) is used to reduce depression and anxiety.
- Tegretol (Carbamazepine) is used to treat severe aggression.
- Trilepal (Oxcarbazepine) is used to treat severe aggression.
- Zoloft (Sertraline) is used to reduce depression and anxiety.

Sleep aids should not be used on a regular basis. Below are the current popular sleep aids that are often prescribed for a person with memory loss:

- Ambien (Zolpidem)
- Lunesta (Eszopiclone)
- Sonata (Zaleplon)

Anti-anxiety medication is used to help people relax and calm agitation. Know that these medications can cause sleepiness, falls, and confusion:

- Ativan (Lorazepam)
- Klonapin (Clonazepam)

Antipsychotics are the big guns that doctors prescribe to treat mental problems such as aggression, paranoia, hallucinations, or agitation:

- Resperdal (Risperdone)
- Seroquel (Quetiapine)
- Zyprexa (Olanzapine)

Medication is not the only answer. Over the years, thousands of clients and their caregivers who have met with me or attended my seminars have learned a different way to deal with difficult behaviors and how to handle them with little or no medication. In many situations, all that is needed are some environmental changes and caregiver education, as well as support to help you the caregiver deal with the challenging behaviors that you may encounter when dealing with the person who has dementia. As you will learn in the next chapters, as the caregiver, sometimes the best medication is education.

CHAPTER FIVE

YOUR PERSPECTIVE AS A CAREGIVER

Before you can deal with any behavior successfully, you'll need to understand yourself and your relationship with the person who has dementia. Dealing with relationships is a learned behavior. Relationships are formed during our lives and are based on expectations, emotions, and capability. No two relationships are alike. As much as we would like to have the same rules apply to everybody, the reality is that different relationships call for different expectations. How you first deal with dementia will be based on your old behavior patterns dealing with this person in the past. If certain things annoyed or drove you crazy in the past, they are going to annoy and drive you crazier now. As a caregiver, you will need to learn better ways to communicate. Let me say this again, and I hope that as a caregiver you will take in what I am saying: the person who has memory loss may look the same and, at times, may act the same, but because of changes in their brain, they are no longer the same.

Often a behavior problem begins because we need the person to be who they once were. This will allow us to continue on with our life as we know it. The person with dementia will have their own way of dealing with a situation that allows them to maintain their individual sense of self and control. Behavior problems often start as an emotional tug of war. You want one thing to happen, and they want another.

Each of you have expectations and want to get your needs met. At some point, it will become impossible for them to be the person they once were, and without knowledge and awareness about this disorder, it will be difficult for you to accept that this is who they are today. But there are ways you can and will get through these moments.

Lesson One: *What Is a Behavior Problem?*

A behavior problem is anything that will cause you, the caregiver, to feel upset, unsure, insecure, or at a loss how to deal with the current situation. Because of your lack of knowledge of dealing with this unfamiliar behavior, you may lash out. You have your own expectations. When those expectations are not met, you may naturally feel anger, frustration, depression, or anxiety. Your past history with the person you are caring for will have an emotional impact on how you deal with them today. You may have unfinished emotional business that you never resolved. Maybe Mom or Dad was emotionally distant or, at the other extreme, too close. As a spouse, you might have stayed in a relationship that years ago you wanted to get out of. Now you may feel trapped.

Behavioral problems will come and go. No behavior will last forever. As a caregiver and a dementia expert I have found only a few behaviors that are cause for concern. Any behavior that puts the person or you in harm's way, threatening your or their safety or life, is a cause for alarm. Behaviors such as aggressiveness, hallucinations, delusions, and wandering can put you or your loved one at risk. Some of these behaviors will need immediate medical or environmental changes. Once again, when in doubt, call 911.

Lesson Two: *Five Steps Toward Solving a Problem Behavior*

1. Isolate the behavior. It is here that you will need to define the problem that is driving you crazy. Is it the repetitive questioning, slowness of getting dressed or eating, aggressive behavior (either physical or verbal), wandering, lack of motivation, hallucinations, agitation, or anxiety that is driving you crazy? Some people become hypersexual, childlike, or over demanding. The most important step that you will take to solve a behavior is to identify the behavior that is causing you the most distress. Next, ask yourself if the behavior is causing distress to the person who is having memory problems. If so, environmental or behavioral changes may be needed. Short-term medication may be necessary.

2. Identify the triggers. The first rule of dementia care is to rule out any medical problem that can be causing this behavior. Could they have a urinary tract infection, fever, depression, dehydration, or pneumonia? Are they in pain that they might not be able to tell you about? After you have ruled out any medical reason for a behavioral problem, you will need to explore possible environmental problems. Some behaviors may be caused by over- or under stimulation, which will cause frustration, boredom, excessive sleeping, depression, aggressiveness, or anger. Grieving and fearful thoughts will cause anxiety. A person who has memory loss will no longer be able to deal rationally with their emotions. A sense of loneliness, abandonment, or a lack of social support can trigger a difficult behavior in some people. Being in situations with too many people

or with new people or in an unfamiliar environment may cause an undesirable reaction.

3. Look for warning signs. Is there a pattern to the behavior? For some people, a certain time of day or a particular season can have an effect on a person with dementia. Too much sleep or lack of sleep will send a person with dementia into a meltdown. The way that your react to a person with dementia—your facial expressions, word choice, and tone of voice—will have an impact on their behavior.

4. Figure out what makes the behavior worse. Anything that a person with dementia believes is attacking their sense of security will make a behavior worse. This can include any change in environment, temperature, or routine. Trying to make a person with dementia do something they do not want to do will make a behavior worse. Trying to rush a person through a task will escalate an unwanted reaction. Remember, you cannot reason with a person who has dementia. Reasoning will make a behavior worse.

5. Figure out what reduces or improves the behavior. Refocus your priorities. As simple as this may sound, refocusing is one thing you can do to successfully deal with a difficult behavior. Your goal is to help the person with dementia feel safe and secure. Constantly telling them what they need to do because it is what they have always done in the past is not only going to defeat your purpose but also going to be frustrating for them. And it will be upsetting to you. This dual frustration is a major cause for most difficult behaviors. What will lessen or improve a behavior? Avoid any form of

confrontation or ordering a person to do something. Keep to a normal routine and familiar people. Learn how to divert an unwanted behavior—with an activity or with food, for example.

Any unrealistic expectations on your part can start a behavioral problem. Expecting a person to do something they once did but can no longer do may trigger an unwanted reaction. Always remember that you are dealing with a person who has lived a full life with a personality of their own. This person, despite the changes in their brain, is still there.

Lesson Three: *Understanding So-Called Difficult Behaviors*

There is no such thing as a difficult behavior. What is difficult is that you have never experienced this problem before. The behavior isn't difficult; you just lack understanding of it. Let's face facts: Everything in life is difficult until you learn how to handle it. From riding a bicycle, swimming, and cooking to dating, knitting, or golfing; everything new is difficult because we've never done it before. With guidance and practice, as you master the steps, it gets easier.

Let's go back to the concept of "difficult." When you label someone or something "difficult," it creates additional problems. You have mentally gone to the word "impossible," which really means "never happening in this lifetime." For caregivers this is often an automatic, unconscious response. So from here on out, every behavior that the person has will be labeled as "difficult." As a caregiver you may lose your focus, and eventually your effectiveness. When you label a behavior "difficult, "what you really mean is that the person you are dealing with is difficult for you to deal with now. But while their current behavior may be difficult for you to manage, it may be easier for someone else to handle.

A person who has dementia is not intentionally "being difficult"; they are just trying to make sense of their world as their brain changes. As a caregiver you want that person to be the same person you've always known. Anything they now do out of their "normal routine" that causes you extra work, stress, or anxiety will be termed "difficult." Instead of difficult behaviors, I prefer to use the term "challenging behaviors": difficult equals hard; challenging equals success. Once you change the way you think, from facing a *difficult* situation to facing a *challenging* situation, you have freed your mind and opened your brain up to new and novel ideas.

There is no such thing as a difficult behavior. The behavior your loved one is now demonstrating is a challenging behavior. The person with dementia will have new behaviors that are going to challenge you. To be a successful caregiver, you will need to learn all you can about this disease and to find new ideas and adapt to new tools that will help both of you maintain a sense of normalcy.

Lesson Four: *Your Expectations and Their Effect*

Many of the behavior problems of a person with dementia are rooted in the caregiver's unrealistic beliefs and expectations. Even though the person with dementia may look the same, the changes in their brain now make them incapable of continuing to fulfill their normal role in the relationship. Labeling this person "difficult" because they are no longer able to continue doing what they have always done is actually an unreasonable expectation. You are setting up yourself and the person with dementia for failure. It's a lose-lose situation. Nobody wins.

A person who has a form of dementia will continue to try to hold on to their previous life even though they are no longer capable of doing so. As a caregiver, you too will try to hold on to your previous life. But as time moves on, so will this disease. If you still expect or want the person with dementia to do what they have always done, you are being unrealistic. It's no longer about them; it's about you and your expectations. The person with dementia is not the only one who is being unreasonable and difficult; you are too. When you hold tightly to the past and continue to expect things to go on as they always have, it makes you and your expectations the problem.

There will be times or moments that you as a caregiver will need to set aside your own innate sense of survival, your own wants and needs. You will need to put the needs of others first and your own needs on the back burner for awhile. To be a successful caregiver, you cannot have it all or do it all. There are only so many hours in the day. If you decide to be a hands-on caregiver, you will have to put your life on hold for the time being and focus on the needs of the person with dementia. When trying to cope with challenging behaviors, you should keep in mind the following facts:

1. A person who has dementia (depending on their stage) may not have the capacity to fully understand the reason or implication of a desired outcome. They might not always have the ability to process the information that is necessary to make a good decision.

2. A person with dementia will avoid danger. Anything that is out of their sense of "normal" is considered dangerous and is to be avoided at all costs. Anything out of their normal routine will threaten their sense

of survival. This includes social events, doctor's appointments, and vacations.

3. A person who has dementia lives in the here and now. The "now" moment is all that matters. Their current needs will have to be met for them to be comfortable.

4. For the person with dementia, there is no longer a future. The changes in their brain cannot register, manage, or imagine future events. Future events cease to exist.

5. People with dementia live in the past. Actually, the past mixes in with the present and becomes the "now." They may no longer recognize you because in the past you didn't exist as you are today. To them, current family members now resemble past or deceased relatives. There will come a time when they look in the mirror and see a stranger. And there will come a time when they no longer recognize you.

As a caregiver, you have choices. As the disease progresses, the window of choice for the person with dementia will slowly close. It is now a struggle between the caregiver, who wants a normal life, and the person with dementia, who is trying to hold on to their normal life. No matter what your relationship is, you have two options: educating yourself as to how to deal with this new situation or walking away. If you choose to stay, learning new tools to deal with this now "new" person is going to be a leap of faith. You can do this.

Eighty percent of my caregiver clients are successful in educating themselves and coping with their loved ones' challenging behaviors. Twenty percent walk away. The majority of those who walk away are the grown children, especially those in the "sandwich" generation; for a few, the reason is past physical or verbal abuse from the person who now has dementia. These cases are rare. Many times grown children walk away because of a misguided sense of their personal entitlement. Many move on in life and no longer feel any obligation to their parents. There is also a group of children who feel that because a sibling is caring for their parent, they have no reason to be financially or emotionally responsible for their parent. I also know spouses who walked away from a partner with dementia. Some spouses prematurely institutionalize their loved one or send them to live with another family member. The reality is that not everyone is able or capable to be caregiver.

Lesson Five: *Changing Your Mind-Set*

No matter what you have encountered in your life, successfully caring for a person who has dementia will likely be the most challenging experience you ever have. No matter what level the person with dementia is currently in, as a caregiver you may feel discomfort, anger, frustration, anxious, and/or depressed. Dealing with a person who has dementia can be challenging and daunting for you. When dealing with challenging behaviors, keep in mind the following points:

1. The person who has a challenging behavior is not always the problem. The problem may be you because you do not understand how to deal with this new side of their personality or behavior.

2. Your behavior will have an effect on the person with dementia. If you get upset, this may cause the person with dementia to become agitated, angry, or

embarrassed. A person with dementia will follow or mimic your emotions.

3. Determine what it is that you want to happen. What is your purpose? Question yourself. Since you know that the person's brain has changed, is changing, and will continue to change, are your expectations reasonable?

4. Forget the past. Don't get upset when the person doesn't operate according to their previous principles or adhere to the principles you think they should adhere to.

5. Slip into the world of the person with dementia. What would you want someone to do for you if you had memory loss?

Lesson Seven: *Understanding What You Are Taking On*

It all comes down to capability. Some caregivers may at first feel doomed. Others may feel a sense of purpose, while still others may be totally paralyzed and have no idea what to make of this new situation. As a caregiver, your feelings and obligations may change overtime. Taking care of a person with dementia will take a toll on your professional, personal, emotional, and financial life, and you should do periodic checkups with yourself to reevaluate how you feel and what you are currently capable of.

Some caregivers will remain stoic no matter how it affects their personal, emotional, or financial present or future. There will be some who will sacrifice all of their time for the person with dementia. There is no way to change their current caregiver mind-set, but I have found that any person who will sacrifice their own time for another person has a personal reason. If you choose to become a caregiver, you know what these reasons are. When my father asked me to care for Mom, I had no idea and (neither did he) what that would mean. Twenty-three years ago, a person with dementia had a ten-year lifespan from the time of diagnosis. Times have changed. Medical interventions and drugs now prolong a person's life. When I first became my mother's caregiver, I had no clue about dementia or how caring for her would change my world. Now I do. Before any person becomes elected by the family or chooses to become a caregiver, the following information needs to be understood.

1. Dementia is a progressive, irreversible brain disorder. Over time, the person who has dementia will need total care. This means around-the-clock, hands-on care because they are no longer able to take care of their daily needs such as bathing, grooming, toileting, transferring, feeding, etc., without help. This is just the physical side of their care. They will also be dependent on you to handle and arrange for their finances, grocery shopping, travel, and activities. The daily list goes on. Caring for a person who has dementia will be a full-time job. You can't do it alone and will need help. Many caregivers rarely ask for help from friends, family, or neighbors. This is a mistake because people may help if asked.

2. Caring for a person who has dementia will cause isolation. There is a stigma associated with dementia. Friends and family may feel that if they are involved with the person with dementia they will somehow "catch" it. Some people are misinformed and think that dementia is contagious. Because of your additional caregiving responsibilities, you may stop

accepting social invitations from friends and family. People will watch you and take their cue from you. If you say, "This is a horrible situation," why would anyone in their right mind want to get involved? The more invitations you turn down, the more you will reinforce to other people the negative perception of what it is like to care for a person who has dementia. The more you isolate yourself and don't ask for help, the more you give people who would like to support you a reason not to help.

3. Do not compare yourself to others. The person you now care for is totally different from individuals you or other people have ever cared for in the past. What techniques previously worked for others in the past may not work well for the person you are now caring for. I have many clients who live in buildings where a lot of the residents have spouses with some form of dementia. They all give each other advice. Often their well-intentioned advice hurts more than it helps. Remember that even though two people are dealing with loved ones who have dementia, their experiences will be different. Even though the diagnosis is the same, you and your loved one are in a unique situation.

CHAPTER SIX

COMMUNICATING WITH A PERSON WHO HAS DEMENTIA

Most behavioral problems of people with dementia are actually a result of a failure to communicate. What makes us unique as individuals is our ability to verbally or physically communicate our needs, wants, and desires. Communication helps us to be understood and to understand another person. As humans, we communicate by language. Language is not always verbal; sometimes it is physical—what we might call body language.

Parents of newborn babies are often stressed out because no matter what they do, they can't always meet their baby's needs. The baby is in misery, and so are their parents. Babies have distinctive vocalizations to express their needs. As a new parent, if you learn to pay close attention and listen carefully, you will recognize that your child has a very specific cry for hunger, diaper change, pain, or separation anxiety. Babies cry because they are not capable of forming words. Just because they cannot speak does not mean that they are not capable of expressing their emotions. A baby's goal is to have their needs met. As most parents of babies quickly learn, if you guess correctly and meet their needs, the crying will stop. For every moment that you fail to meet their needs, the baby's anxiety kicks up a notch or two; sometimes, even when you finally figure out what was wrong and correct it, you don't know if you've met their needs because the baby continues to cry. The crying often starts out of frustration, pain, or discomfort; the crying continues because once the roller coaster of anxiety starts, it's hard to stop. This same roller coaster holds true for a person with dementia.

To effectively deal with a person who is having any form of memory loss, the first step is to get a good diagnosis so that you will have an understanding of what you and the person you are caring for are now dealing with. The next step is to become an effective communicator. Being able to communicate effectively is the most important aspect of caring for a person with dementia.

Lesson One: *Understanding the Effects of Communication Problems*

Communication includes not just spoken language but body language, tone of voice, and eye contact. When you are dealing with a person who has dementia, as they progress through the stages of the disease, words will lose their importance, and body language, tone of voice, and eye contact will become important.

Because of their memory loss, a person with dementia will have problems finding, retrieving, or recalling the word they want to use. It is due to their word-finding problems that they have difficulty expressing their thoughts, needs, wants, and desires. Because of their memory and concentration loss, they have a shortened attention span. This will make it harder for them to follow conversations or to understand what you ask them to do. They have lost the ability to make sense out of long conversations or explanations, or they are no longer able to complete a set of tasks when given verbal instructions. As the dementia progresses, you will need to change the way you communicate in order to help the person with dementia understand you. There will come a time when a person will go from complete understanding of your request to just being able to understand the first three words that you say and then to only being able to follow simple one-word commands.

The less a person is able to verbally communicate, the more they will now rely on facial and body expressions to explain to them what is happening. This just means that a person with dementia who has lost their ability to speak will now rely on your gestures, tone of voice, physical touch, and voice volume to communicate. Your body and facial language speaks volumes to a person with dementia. I often say that people with dementia have a sixth sense. As the disease progresses, the person with dementia becomes more sensitive to other people's body language than ever before. Like a person who is blind, the person with dementia who is having a problem with verbal communication will become more sensitive to other forms of communication, namely facial and body movements. The tone of voice from the person who is speaking becomes important. A person with dementia is hypersensitive to the facial expressions, tone of voice, and body language of other people. Remember that a person who has dementia is confused, anxious, and fearful; they are seeking the safety of the familiar. This is where a good understanding of communication is important. Communication is not just about what we say but how we say it—our communication style—which includes tone, facial expressions, and body language.

When you are dealing with a person who has dementia, you are now dealing with a person who is no longer capable of following the rules. I will use a boxing ring analogy to explain. I am not a fan of boxing (blows to the head can cause dementia), but boxing does give some insight into the world of communication and communication styles. For a match, boxers are paired according to their weight class, which gives each opponent an opportunity to win. Having a person who weighs 180 pounds boxing in the same ring with a person who weighs 130 pounds would not be fair. This is why boxers are placed in classes of weight: light, middle, and heavy. No one in their right mind would pair a lightweight with a heavyweight in the same ring.

Because of the changes to their brain, people with dementia are no longer in the same mental weight class. Remember, they may look the same, sound the same, and— at times—act the same, but they really are not the same. As the person with dementia progresses through this disease, you will remember how to fight by the rules, and they will not. So say good-bye to fair fights. As the disease progresses, the person caring for a person with dementia will be at a disadvantage. And with additional education and understanding, both of you can make it through this time and find new ways to communicate with each other.

Communication problems happen to the best of us, even those of us who are experts in the field. Past problems that have gone unresolved continue through today. In my office, I see families who have past hurts they never overcame, and they will use today to "right a wrong" at a time when the other person is no longer able to. I have adult children in my office who will lash out, disconnect from the situation, or become the perfect child to deal with problems from their past. When it comes to communication you should also know that past pain, anger, frustration, regret, or despair that wasn't addressed or dealt with may now come out as a behavioral issue. How you approach these unresolved problems will affect how you communicate with a person who has dementia.

Lesson Two: *Making Communication More Effective*

Understanding communication styles is a big business. Lawyers often hire communication experts to help them in jury selection, to observe how the trial is going, and to gauge the reactions of the jury. The lawyers receive feedback as to how the jury is doing and which jurors the lawyers should pay attention to in order to win the case. It would be a wonderful world if all caregivers could hire a communication expert to come into our home to help us understand the person we are now caring for.

People who have word-finding problems may also have difficulty with reading as well as communicating with others. You may be speaking the same language, but the meaning isn't always the same. In short, the message a person is trying to send out needs to be validated. If the communication is properly received, the person feels good, and if it's not, they may become anxious, frustrated, or angry. This is where communication and behavioral problems happen. To be an effective communicator you will need to be a good observer.

To be an observer may mean that you will need to back away from the moment. You will need to choose the right words, pay close attention to what is happening, keep your train of thought, and diminish background distractions. It will also help if you are able to keep your personal frustration to a minimum, especially if the communication isn't working.

There are times that communication is affected by past hurts. As a therapist, I often help families deal with past injuries and to successfully help them let go of the past. Through therapy, we deal with the past and move beyond the anger or hurt, in order to deal with the now. If the person with dementia is able, and you as a caregiver are willing to deal with difficult emotions, this may open up a deeper level of communication between you and the person you are now caring for. Through years of clinical practice I have discovered that individual counseling is effective for those who are in the mild stages of dementia. Just because a person has short-term memory loss doesn't mean what happened in the past is forgotten. In fact, long-term memory stays intact for years. Therapy can help to reduce some behaviors. My practice is filled with caregivers who want to be better caregivers, and through therapy they are able to do so. How? As we work through the steps of learning about dementia, we also deal with past and current family issues. As a caregiver, making peace with yesterday may allow you to successfully move on and become a better caregiver today.

Lesson Three: *The Role of Family Dynamics*

Any person who was physically, sexually, or emotionally abused in the past by the person with dementia and is now the caregiver will have a particularly difficult time with their caregiver role. Without proper guidance or therapy, all I can say is, "Good luck." In many families, elder abuse is a reality. Take a vulnerable elder, and place them under the care of a person who has a past grudge: this is often a recipe for disaster. Family dynamics are not understood by many professionals and are either discounted or overlooked when a family first consults a doctor. As a professional therapist, I'm able to spot these problems in a heartbeat.

I received a phone call recently from a person who was referred to me from another agency. Jane was upset because her mother, whom she has always been close to, now "hated her." No matter what Jane did, Mom kept her at a distance, rejected her, and resented her help. Jane was upset. Up until two years ago, she and her mother had a good relationship with each other. Then Jane's mom started changing. She became emotionally distant, reclusive, and argumentative. As I began to explore Jane's relationship with her mother, she started to take her anger out on me. Calmly, I asked about her mother's relationships with other family members. According to Jane, everything was fine. I kept asking questions, and she remembered that Mom actually hated her sister (Jane's aunt) because she was mean to their mother when they were growing up. Because of memory loss, Mom had confused her daughter with her sister. Once Jane came to understand that her mother wasn't upset with her but with her sister, Jane was able to successfully deal with the situation and continue to care for her mother.

Spouses often have an intimate form of communication that may change over time, depending on the degree of dementia. I know couples who loved to banter but now no longer can. I also know couples whose main form of communication was arguing, but now their loved one is no longer able to. I have clients who normally would playfully pinch or touch one another. This is how their relationships developed and continued. Once a person has dementia, they may no longer be able to understand this previous form of communication.

When it comes to anyone over sixty-five, conversations about sex are the least talked-about change, but one that can cause significant relationship problems. When it comes to dealing with spouses, especially those who have had a close physical/sexual relationship in the past, memory issues are not their major concern; the loss of physical intimacy is. At this time you or the person you are caring for may feel abandoned, rejected, or hurt. It may help to talk about your concerns with a therapist.

A major caregiver concern I often hear is that the caregiver made a promise that they are now not able to keep. One of my biggest challenges is helping caregivers resolve this dilemma. Caregivers are often asked by a family member or the person they are caring for to promise that they will never be placed in a nursing home. In the long run, this promise may not be in the best interest of the person they are caring for.

Years ago my father made me promise that I would care for my mother at home no matter what. I agreed. Later on he was hospitalized, and placed on the same floor with a person who had dementia. After listening to the screaming and moaning for three days (and so did I after visiting him for twelve hours a day), my father changed his position on Mom's care. After he was discharged from the hospital, my father told me that he was sorry that he had made me promise to care for my mother at home and made me promise instead that if Mom's behavior affected me or my family, I would place her in a facility. I'm not going to lie and say that I wasn't thrilled that I was off the hook and could place my mother in a facility without guilt if her care became overwhelming or difficult for me. Knowing that I now had the option gave me the freedom to choose the best place for my mother's care.

When it comes to dealing with a person who has dementia, you have to know yourself and what you are capable of handling. Forget about what you may have promised in the past. That promise was made in a time of good faith, manipulation, guilt, or emotional pressure. It may be better for all parties if the promise that you made is broken. Daily care for a person with memory loss will be disruptive and will change your life. Caring for a person who has any form of dementia is not going to be easy. To be a good caregiver, you will need to be honest with yourself.

Lesson Four: *How Dementia Affects Communication*

At some point, because of the changes to their brain, a person with dementia may experience:

- limited vocabulary
- lapses in train of thought
- changes in orientation (being able to know time and place)
- changes to the five senses
- revert to using their first language

Over time, a person with dementia will eventually lose their ability to remember familiar words. They may and often will substitute words, use inappropriate words, or use simple words to get their needs met. They may also make up new words to express themselves. As the disease progresses, their vocabulary will become basic. Instead of a shower they may say "bath"; "eat" replaces lunch or dinner; going to the mall becomes "going out." They use short phrases to convey what they want or what they need. As they lose vocabulary skills, they may make up new words or expressions that will make sense to them, but maybe not to you or other people who are close to them. If there comes a time when you can't figure out what it is that they want or what they are trying to express, this may lead to frustration and anxiety for both of you. Because of their declining vocabulary they will become repetitive. For the caregiver, the constant repeating of questions or phrases is annoying. For the person with dementia, repetition is a comfort.

A person who has dementia will have difficulty with their ability to think and process information, which will cause a lapse in their train of thought. Because of this lapse, they will have a difficult time engaging in a conversation or being able to remain focused on a specific task. Memory loss also affects a person's ability to reason, use judgment, perceive, and understand. As a caregiver you will need to focus on the person who has dementia and constantly redirect and guide them to stay on task. With your help and guidance, a person with dementia will be able to continue to be involved in conversations and activities that will help them remain independent for a longer period.

At birth, our brains are wired with five main senses: touch, smell, taste, hearing, and sight. For most of us, aging will compromise some of the five senses. This is the reason that many people will have additional problems, besides dementia, that will need to be addressed. As we age, our sense of touch may become less or more sensitive. Arthritis will affect our joints and make a common task or a favorite hobby, such as knitting, difficult to do. Once nimble fingers may now find it difficult to use a zipper or button a shirt. As a result of body changes or accidents, many older people will have problems with their knees or feet that will make walking painful or make it difficult to stand (which may make some people more prone to falls). As people age, it is natural for their sense of smell and taste to be reduced. This is why some people might not recognize that food they are served is spoiled or that there's something burning in the kitchen.

As people age, their taste buds become less sensitive. Food tastes different, so they may need to add more spices because their taste buds are not sending signals to the brain. Their sense of the temperature of food is no longer accurate. Food is either too hot or too cold. Some people will have mouth problems caused by their dentures (which can block taste) or periodontal problems, which will cause food to taste different. In some people, a trauma to the head may cause a change to their sense of smell and taste.

As people age, their vision will also change. My vision was perfect up until I was sixteen years old. Then I needed glasses. Over the years my vision has changed, and without glasses or contact lenses, things look blurry. Recently because of allergies and perhaps falling asleep one too many times with my contact lenses in, my corneas became scratched, and I was forced to wear trifocal glasses instead of contact lenses.

I got dizzy wearing the trifocals and had trouble driving and walking. Stairs were an obstacle. Since I've always had a depth perception problem, driving and parking the car for me was a challenge. I also had bruises (and a few broken toes) from all the doorways, walls, and furniture that I bumped into. When I wore glasses, I limited my activities. I stopped participating in sports. I wore single-vision lenses for distance and then used reading glasses to do my work. I got nauseous and dizzy. Meals were even worse. If I didn't wear my reading glasses, the food was a blur; if I wore my reading glasses, socialization was a blur.

I lost weight and reduced socialization with my coworkers because of vision problems. Food was no longer appetizing, and socializing without seeing faces was exhausting and unappetizing. Everyone in my office whom I socialize with speaks Spanish; for me to understand any language I need to see their faces and gestures. Without good vision, I withdrew from friends, family, coworkers, and food. Needless to say, because of my vision problems, I became depressed.

Once I got the okay from my eye doctor to start using my contact lenses again, my life returned to normal. Food now looks and tastes good, I no longer bang into walls or furniture (okay, occasionally I still do—contact lenses can only do so much), and I once again actively participate in life. As a caregiver you need to know that a change in a person's vision will affect their appetite, socialization, and motivation. Loss of vision can cause depression. Depression will affect memory.

For some of us, aging may cause our hearing to diminish. Not to point out the obvious, but you cannot remember what you do not hear. Men in particular have a difficult time accepting using any form of hearing aid. They may use a walker or cane, wear glasses, have prostrate problems, and use Viagra, but they refuse to use a hearing aid. Go figure! Many of the clients I see have a hearing problem, which is the cause of what appears to be a memory problem. Trust me, get the person fitted with a good hearing aid that they can and will use, and their memory will most likely improve.

We live in a world of many languages. Over 50 percent of my clients are bilingual. Many of my older clients met their spouses during World War II, the Vietnam War, or the Cuban boat lift, or they come from Haiti, Mexico, or South America. They fell in love with someone whose first language was not English or who didn't speak their primary language. Any person who has dementia will revert back to using their native language. Even if this person did learn a new language and used it well for years, they will revert back to their original language from birth or their first few years of life. If you are not fluent in their native language, you are going to be at a loss.

Lesson Five: *Twelve Steps to Better Communication*

The following steps should help make communication between you and the person with dementia easier.

1. Always focus your full attention on them. Turn off the radio or television. Do not talk on the phone in front of them. Avoid any distractions. Keep eye contact,

remain patient, and, most importantly, try to listen to their wants and needs.

2. Use feelings instead of facts. The person with dementia may have a hard time describing what it is that they want. You may need to listen to their feelings and body language to determine what it is they need or are trying to explain.

3. Use a familiar name. As the person with dementia "time travels," depending on when and where in time they think they are, a familiar name may help orient them. Many of my clients are in their second, third, or fourth marriage. If you use their current last name, this may cause anxiety because they have no clue who that person is. I noticed that when I greeted my mother, who in severe end-stage dementia, with "Hi Mom," she'd flinch. In her current stage of this disease, my mother no longer could recognize or conceive that she is my mother. When I greeted her with "Hi Katie" (her childhood name), she no longer flinched and instead smiled at me.

4. Turn questions into answers. Do not ask a person with dementia if they have to go to the bathroom. Instead say, "Let's go to the bathroom." The same goes for bathing or eating. Do not ask if they would like to take a bath or eat. The person with dementia will usually say no. Direct them to what needs to be done.

5. Do not quiz a person who has dementia. Try not to use the word "remember." You are dealing with a person who has a memory problem—encounters should not be a game show moment. When looking through the family album or pictures on the wall, don't ask, "Who

are these people?" Pick up or point to the picture and say, "You have a beautiful family. Tell me about them." Let the person with dementia take the lead.

6. Ask them to do one task at a time. Too many directions given at one time can be confusing and overwhelming for a person with dementia. You will need to break down each task into simple steps. Instead of telling a person with dementia to get out of bed, take a shower, get dressed, and come down for breakfast, you will need to focus on one task at a time. You may need to help the person with dementia take a shower, lay out their clothes to help them dress, and then escort them to the breakfast table.

7. Be careful how you speak. Try not to use words that can be taken out of context. Because of their now limited vocabulary, if you tell a person to "hop into the shower," they may try to hop or realize that they can't hop and will resist showering. I had a caregiver who, when her mother said that she had to go to the bathroom, told her to "Go now." The person with dementia told her daughter three times that she had to go to the bathroom. Each time the daughter kept saying, "Go now." Well, she finally did; the daughter was mortified, and Mom was embarrassed because she urinated on the couch. A person with dementia will take what you say literally. Had the daughter said, "Mom, let's go to the bathroom," and taken her, this situation would have been avoided.

8. Be specific. Instead of asking a person where they put "it," ask, for example, where they put the house keys. Remember that you are dealing with a person

who has short-term memory loss. If they are looking for something that is misplaced, keep naming the misplaced item to keep the person with dementia on track and on task for what they are trying to find.

9. Always treat people with dignity and respect. I used to say to caregivers to treat their loved ones as they would want their parents to be treated. The reality is that some parents were not the greatest. I now use the golden rule: "Treat others how you would like to be treated."

10. Use a gentle, relaxed tone. A person with dementia will pick up and mirror your reaction. They will look to you for behavioral clues and for guidance. If your tone is gentle and relaxed, they will mirror your behavior. If you are stressed out and unnerved, this too will be mirrored.

11. Keep your message short. Remember the acronym K.I.S.S.: Keep It Simple and Short. You will have to change your current way of communicating that is no longer working and learn to keep your sentences short. Instead of saying, "Honey, tonight we are going to dinner with the Smiths, and remember that he likes to talk about golf," try saying first, "We are eating with the Smiths." Later add in the "golf" portion. Break it down into small parts: Dinner, Smiths, golf.

12. Use touch. Our sense of touch helps to validate who we are and keeps us focused. Touch is a nonverbal form of communication that conveys warmth and caring to some. Know who you are touching. I enjoy using touch and being touched, but some people hate to be

touched. Learn to respect and accept another person's personal boundaries.

13. Keep your sense of humor. If you are caring for a person who enjoys humor, keep the jokes coming. When a person does something that is funny, laugh about what happened instead of criticizing them. Humor can defuse a challenging behavior.

Final Thoughts on Communication

Dealing with a person who has dementia is not easy. If you follow the steps listed above, it will help make both of your lives easier. Here are some additional tips, based on my experience with my clients and personally, that I have found to be very useful:

1. Do not try to argue or reason with the person who has dementia. Not only will you lose, but they will become combative and/or anxious. Think of a two-year-old in a grocery store who wants candy: a total meltdown. Instead, validate the needs of the person you are caring for, and divert their attention elsewhere.

2. A person with dementia is anxious because they are unsure of what is expected of them. Assure them that you will be there for them in a calm and soothing voice.

3. People who have dementia will be repetitive. This is just a stage, but it can be emotionally exhausting to the caregiver. It's like taking a road trip to Disney World with a three-year-old who keeps saying over and over and over again, "Are we there yet?" For me, this is beyond annoying. My gut reaction after the

twentieth time is to smack the little bugger (but I have self-control, so I don't, but I really, really want to!). The reality is that a person who has dementia will be repetitive because they are anxious. They know that there is somewhere they are supposed to be, and they want to be there on time because this is what they have been programmed by societal values to do. At this stage, a person with dementia still cares about going to an event or being on time. As annoying as the repetition is, be happy that the person is still involved. As the dementia progresses, your loved one will lose interest in being an active participant or will lose their vocabulary and no longer ask. You may later wish to have back those moments of "Are we there yet?" Try to reassure the person with dementia, and use a calming voice to respond to whatever they ask.

4. Once again, try not to ask a person who has any form of memory disorder if they "remember" something. Their memory is impaired. If they could remember, they and you wouldn't be in this situation. Playing any form of game show questioning is not going to bring back their memory. It will only cause a person with dementia to have anxiety, feel bad, and withdraw or lash out. Instead, reminisce about the past, and try to draw the person with dementia into the current conversation.

5. Try not to use the phrase "You can't . . ." Encourage the person who has dementia to do as much as they are able to do. Be aware of their current physical and cognitive limitations, and do not ask them to do anything that is out of their realm. The person may no longer be able to cook dinner, but they can still

(with some direction) help with the salad or set the table. Everybody wants to be useful. Give step-by-step instructions. As their dementia progresses, they may no longer be able to do all of the steps that it takes to wash and dry a load of laundry independently, but they are still capable of doing small steps, such as picking clothes out of the hamper, sorting by color, placing them into the washing machine, or transferring the washed clothes into the dryer. Even if someone is confined to a bed, you should still try to engage them and give them an opportunity to help out. Give them towels or clothes to fold. Everyone gets joy out of feeling useful and contributing to the family or the household.

Keep in mind that just because a person with dementia may have difficulty in one area of their life does not mean that they will have difficulty in all areas. Good communication will mean being aware of the problems a person with dementia has and then helping them get through the situation.

CHAPTER SEVEN

COPING WITH CHANGES IN DAILY LIFE

As time goes on, a person who has dementia will find it difficult to successfully pay their bills, cook, shop alone for food or clothes, remember important appointments or dates such as doctor's appointments or important events such as birthdays or holidays, continue with their hobbies, or make travel plans. There will come a time when they will forget to take or will stop taking their medication. They may refuse to take medication. Most caregivers miss recognizing these moments. The progression of this disease is usually so slow that many people do not notice the subtle changes in their loved ones, especially when they see them day in and day out. For caregivers who live far away, the reassuring phone call puts their minds at ease. Another reason that caregivers may miss out on changes is that the person they care for has always been responsible, so they naturally assume that if the person is still doing or seems capable of doing what they once did, then all is well. Then there are those (including doctors) who will attribute any change in self-care, behavior, or forgetfulness to normal aging. Another reason that changes in our loved ones often go unaddressed is that admitting there is a problem means that someone will have to deal with the problem. Coming to terms that a loved one has dementia can be overwhelming.

When you are dealing with a person who has any form of dementia, the changes that may be first recognizable to you are in the area of independent activities of daily living (IADLs) or in their activities of daily living (ADLs).

Lesson One: *Understanding IADLs and Their Significance*

IADL are things you and I often take for granted, but they are important because being able to do them allows us to live in society as independent adults. IADLs give us the freedom to plan and execute what we want to do in order to live successfully in today's society. In order to be independent, a person must be capable of doing such things as handling their finances, paying bills, making and keeping doctor's appointments, filling and taking prescribed medication, preparing a meal, making plans with friends, arranging travel arrangements, following a movie, playing a card game, going grocery or clothes shopping, and so on.

If a person is no longer able to pay their bills on time, prepare a meal (or order a delivery meal), or take their medication consistently, or they miss doctor's appointments or social events, then they will need some assistance. If the bills don't get paid, the utilities will be shut off. If they can no longer cook meals, they'll suffer nutritionally, and if they forget to take their medication, they'll become ill. If a person is having trouble remembering appointments and holidays or making travel plans, they will become socially isolated and miss out on important functions. To successfully be independent, a person needs to be able to do the following.

- plan
- procure
- execute

For example, consider a typical dinner. In order to make dinner, there are several steps involved. First, you have to plan the meal (this means envisioning a future occurrence) and decide who and how many people you will be serving, what you are going to serve, and the time that it will take to cook the dinner. The next step is to put together the necessary ingredients. Do you already have what is needed, or will you have to go to the grocery store to get them? Let's assume that you need some additional things that are not in your kitchen. You will make a list and then go shopping. You will need to get to the store. Once in the store, you need to find the item and put it in your cart. If they don't have the items that you need, you might consider changing your original meal to fit what the grocer has. You will also have to be able to pay for the food—to have enough cash or use a credit card. Whether by foot, bus, cab, or car, you will have to get back home. Once home, you will need to unload the groceries that you just bought and put them where they belong. Now comes the fun part: you need to pull together and prepare the meal. This is where you put all of the ingredients together, choose the proper pan, set the correct oven temperature, prepare the side dishes, set the table, take the meal out of the oven, and wait for your guests or spouse to arrive. I do not have any form of dementia that I am aware of, and I have ruined a dinner or two (okay, I've personally ruined several dinners over the past few years). A person who is having memory problems will go far beyond a ruined dinner.

The added stress of preparing a meal will cause many persons with dementia to stop making dinner altogether, and they will excuse themselves from cooking. Many of my clients say things like, "I've made dinners for forty-five years, and I'm tired of cooking," or "It's just your father and me; it's easier to go out." Many spouses will go along with their partner's perspective, and to most family members and friends, this change to their dinner plans will appear normal. Most of us can relate. So the family now rationalizes that Mom is right; after all the years she spent in the kitchen, she deserves a break. For my clients and as an expert on dementia, I will agree: an occasional break from cooking is normal. But retirement from cooking is not. The reality is that a person who has memory loss will (in their quest for normalcy) give really good answers that will make sense unless you know what you are dealing with. The following is a typical conversation with a person with dementia (PWD):

ME: Yes, after cooking all of these years for your family, you definitely deserve a break. So for dinner tonight would you rather order in or eat out?

PWD: It doesn't matter.

ME: Would you rather eat in or eat out?

PWD: Whatever you want is fine with me.

ME: This is about what you want.

PWD: I don't care; anything is fine.

ME: If you could choose any food, what would you eat?

PWD: Anything will be fine with me. You choose.

ME: I want you to have what you want.

PWD: I'm not hungry; you decide.

And so it goes. Actually the above conversation is a typical conversation in my office. A person with dementia often sounds "normal," and what they say and how they respond make sense. The reality is that people with memory loss can and do fake it. The families who get to watch this exchange in my office are amazed. What they once took for granted as being "normal" they now realize is something else. "Normal" Mom used to jump out of bed to make the pancakes from scratch for them or for Dad. For many of my clients, the above exchange is a wake-up call that something is wrong.

Keep in mind, any change in a person's normal behavior is a red flag that something is wrong. If a person once loved to cook and now shows little interest, there is a problem. A person who has memory loss will be able to use the best and most authentic reasons to cover up their memory loss. This is called compensation. As caregivers and family members, we believe their reasoning. Some reasons you may hear are:

- I'm tired of doing the taxes.
- I can't see as well as I used to.
- I've cooked all of my life, and I'm tired of it.
- I don't want to go out with other people; I have nothing in common with them.
- All of my friends have either moved away or died.
- There's nothing good on TV.
- I don't read the paper anymore because it's all bad news.

And the comments go on and on and on. The reasons given sound good and logical. The reality is that most of their reasons are excuses or a cover-up.

As a caregiver, you are now powerless to reverse this situation; however, there are steps you can take to make it better for both you and the person with dementia. Recognize what is happening, and allow the person with dementia to maintain their dignity. Do not force the issue. If you notice that they are having a problem preparing a meal, help them out. If a person is having a problem paying bills, offer to help them. If you notice that they are not taking their medication, gently remind them. Once a person has lost the ability to do their IADLs, there is no turning back. There is no medication or cognitive retraining that will return the person to their previous functioning. What you can offer is support. The support you offer will help the person with memory loss to keep their normal routine. This will allow them to have a sense of independence and feel good about themselves.

Once a person stops doing what they have always done or enjoyed doing, the moment for change or rehabilitation has passed. There is no magic pill or therapy that will return your loved one to their previous independence, but there are things you can do to help them remain independent and to maintain their self-esteem.

1. Hire a financial consultant. When it comes the time where the person with dementia is financially challenged or is no longer able to manage their finances, a good consultant is worth what you pay them. Do not rely simply on word-of-mouth or recommendations. Thoroughly check out the consultant or agency. Contact the Better Business Bureau.

2. Hire a personal driver. The cost of owning a car— once you include the price of gasoline, insurance, and maintenance—can be a luxury in some places. For many people, selling the car is a good and safe decision. This will also reduce their estates exposure to future lawsuits.

3. Sign up for free transportation. Many cities have grants through the state that will provide transportation to those who can no longer drive or have physical or mental disabilities.

4. When you cannot be there, you will need to hire someone to replace you as caregiver. Whether it be medication management, food shopping, or going to a doctor's appointment, if you cannot be there to oversee these things, then make sure that someone else will. If you do not have another family member or friend who can step in, consider hiring a geriatric care manager who as an expert will coordinate care. A geriatric care manager will develop a good care plan and can follow through with their daily needs and reassess as needed to ensure optimal care.

5. Put in a change of address. If you don't live with the person with dementia (or in some cases even if you do), have all of the bills routed to you or a post office box, or pay bills online. The goal is that services such as utilities are continued and important policies like long-term care, health care, and life insurance do not get canceled or changed. Set up automatic bill payments for all the usual bills, such as phone, electricity, and cable television. Consider setting up automatic payments with the newspaper, pool service, mortgage, long-term care insurance, property and vehicle taxes, home insurance, and any other ongoing accounts.

6. If you are concerned about medication management, start using a pill box or medication reminders. If you can, call the person at pill time. Realize that some people may not take their medication no matter what they may tell you. Consider using a service that will call daily to remind the person to take their medication, and have them use an electronic pill dispenser. If

this doesn't work, hire an aide who will visit daily to oversee and give medications.

7. If the person is having any type of memory loss and continues to drive, you should have their driving evaluated. We all consider ourselves to be safe drivers. But a person with memory loss may not recognize that they are having problems driving. Neither will the spouse or family member who needs this person to be independent. My rule of thumb: if you feel uncomfortable putting your children, grandchildren, or neighbor's children in the person's car, now is a good time to reassess the person's driving ability.

8. Most accidents happen at home. In chapter 9, I will help you safety-proof the home. A person with memory loss will forget that they shouldn't climb up a ladder or cook on the stove. The best money you will ever spend is to have a professional evaluate the home and recommend ways to make the home safe now and in the future.

9. Anyone who lives alone or spends time alone should have a personal response system. With a push of a button, help is on the way.

10. Have prepared meals delivered. If a person is not able to cook or has difficulty leaving their home, hire a service or a person to make their meals. Another option is to contact a local restaurant and arrange to have meals delivered to their home. An additional bonus is that these types of services may build a relationship with your loved one and can alert you to changes in behavior.

Lesson Two: *Understanding ADLs and Levels of Independence*

ADLs (activities of daily living) are self-care skills such as toileting, grooming, dressing, feeding, and transferring (moving from one position to another). As adults, if we don't have a physical disability, we are expected to be able to go to the bathroom, shower, eat, and move around by ourselves. If we can do all of these things without help, we are considered to be self-sufficient. When the time comes that a person needs some help with their ADLs, they are no longer considered to be independent. They will now need additional help to get them through their day.

The amount of help the person needs will vary. Care needed is based on the diagnosis, the stage they are in, and their physical and cognitive capabilities. The first level of help is when the person only needs reminders of what needs to be done. Let's use bathing as an example. I call the first level "Honey, it's time to bathe." At this point, a person may only need a verbal reminder to clue them in to what needs to be done. The next level of help is supervision. This is where another person will need to verbally guide the person through the steps of bathing or watch over them when they are taking a shower. The third level is when some hands-on help is required. At this level you will need to guide them to the bathroom and physically help a person in the shower. You may need to help them with the washcloth and soap and verbally guide them through the steps to bathe. The fourth level is when a person is totally dependent on the caregiver. You will need to lead them into the shower and physically bathe them. The fifth level of care is when the person with dementia is chair-or bed-bound and they are totally dependent on you or others to physically bathe them.

The degree of care will vary from one person to another and even change on a daily basis. Keep in mind that just because a person needs some help in some areas does not mean that they are unable to do other things independently for themselves. As the dementia progresses, the level of help they need to successfully accomplish their ADLs will increase. As a caregiver you will need to become more involved in their daily personal care. A person with dementia (and their family) may not recognize that they now need additional help. A rule of thumb for ADLs: when your loved one stays in the same clothes day after day, they need your help.

At some point you may need to answer questionnaires about your loved one's ADLs and IADLs. Most of us fill these forms out based on voluntary self-deception. Answer with this question in mind: Could the person do this on their own without my or another persons help? In my practice I often hear that Mom "never did her taxes." The way to think of the question is, even though she never did her finances, would she be able to contact an accountant and give them the financial information they need? I have many clients who never cooked a meal. If they now needed to, without help, could they put together a meal or call in for delivery? As a caregiver you need to answer the questions honestly.

When it comes to family members, personal care is the biggest concern I hear about. Dad not being able to do his taxes is one thing; Dad not making it to the bathroom is a whole different realm. The rest of this chapter focuses on ADLs and gives you the tools you will need to successfully handle caregiving for a person with dementia in terms of daily activities.

Toileting

Overtime, a person who has dementia will have difficulty recognizing or remembering that they need to go to the bathroom. Actually, they may forget what a bathroom is. The clinical term is "incontinence." Incontinence is the condition in which a person either cannot make it to the bathroom in time or is unaware that they need to use a bathroom. Sometimes incontinence is caused by not being able to locate a bathroom or to understand the purpose of the bathroom. The steps required to remove clothing may be the cause of premature toileting problems. Some people may no longer be able to recognize that they need to use the bathroom, or their body no longer sends or accepts the brain's signal that they have to go to the bathroom. If you notice that your loved one is having a problem with incontinence, these are steps you can take to address it:

1. Make an appointment for the person to see the urologist. You need to rule out any medical condition that can be causing an incontinence problem.

2. Ask the person's doctor if medications might be causing the problem. If a medication is for "calming" a behavior, it may also calm the bladder or bowels.

3. Establish a routine in which you take the person to the bathroom regularly.

4. Limit nighttime fluid intake. A good idea is to have the person stop drinking fluids after 6 PM. You should make sure that the person has enough liquids during the day to reduce dehydration.

5. Place signs to indicate where the bathroom is.

6. Evaluate the person's clothing. Some clothes are easier to remove, such as elastic-waist pants. Trying to unbuckle a belt, unbutton a button, and unzip a pair of pants when the person has an urge to go can cause a toileting accident.

7. Keep a light on in the bathroom.

8. Change the color of the toilet seat. Many bathrooms are one color, and this makes it difficult to distinguish the toilet. Consider changing the colors in the bathroom to make the toilet stand out.

9. If the person is having problems with walking or falling and they are in the beginning stages of dementia, consider purchasing a bedside commode. A person who has mild memory loss may be able to be trained to use this new "toilet."

10. Buy disposable pads for beds, furniture, and your car.

11. Encourage the person to use the bathroom. Do not ask a person if they have to go to the bathroom, simply say, "Let's go to the bathroom," and then take them.

12. Some liquids may have a diuretic effect. If possible, reduce the use of caffeinated beverages such as coffee, tea, soda, or liquor especially in the evening.

Of all behaviors associated with the ADLs, incontinence will be your biggest challenge. Caring for a person who is incontinent is difficult. It's not something you ever envisioned. The twelve steps listed above are some suggestions to try to help with and avoid incontinence. If you have worked through these steps and are still having problems, do not take it personally or feel bad. A person with dementia will eventually lose their ability to recognize the feeling they need to use the bathroom. No one does this on purpose; nobody wants to have an accident. Some of my clients told me that that their roof leaked over their bed, and this is why their bed is wet in the morning. Others have said to me that during dinner or while having a snack they accidentally spilled their drink on their lap. Some people tell me that a stranger came in to use their toilet and missed, or that someone comes in at night and poops on their floor. A few clients tell me that they "might" be having a problem with their bladder or bowels.

When an adult no longer can control their bladder or their bowels, it will cause the caregiver distress. I have clients who now urinate in the kitchen sink, on the floor, in a corner of the bedroom, a closet, or outdoors—sometimes on the front lawn in front of the neighbors. With proper guidance, many of my clients are able to handle bladder incontinence. When my three year old son peed outside, by a tree, neighbors would laugh. When my eighty-year-old mother did the same thing, neighbors freaked out!

Urination is one thing; dealing with the bowels is something else. We aren't prepared to address or deal with bowel problems. We might have had some experience changing diapers for our children or grandchildren, but let's be honest: the thought of changing a diaper for a parent or spouse never crossed our minds. I know this firsthand because for two years I was responsible for changing my father's diapers since Mom had dementia and wasn't able to care for her husband. Needless to say, I am now traumatized. I have PTDD (post traumatic diaper disorder). The physical care of my father, who did not have dementia, became my responsibility, and this meant changing his diapers. After this experience, my family now understands that when it comes to changing diapers for anyone over twenty-five pounds or older than three years old, count me out. Over the past twenty years, I have had the opportunity to speak with thousands of caregivers. Suffice to say that incontinence, especially bowel incontinence, is a major reason why family members place their loved ones in a facility.

Bathing

Bath time is a huge challenge for caregivers. Next to incontinence, this is a major caregiver concern. As a caregiver you will find that over time, a person who has dementia may lose their desire and ability to bathe. Due to the progression of this disease a person with dementia will have several (often valid) reasons as to why they do not need to bathe:

1. They believe that have already bathed; therefore they do not need another bath.

2. They no longer are doing activities that they once did; therefore they don't sweat.

3. Why bathe if they are just going to stay home?

4. They already gave themselves a sponge bath.

5. They are depressed and lack the motivation or desire to bathe.

6. They have forgotten some of the steps to bathing.

7. They have a fear of water.

8. They are afraid of the shower.

9. They have a fear of falling.

10. They do not want to ruin their hairdo.

Let's take some of the above objections to bathing and make some sense of their beliefs. Keep in mind that sometimes the person does have a valid argument.

1. Remember, a person with memory problems will have difficulty recalling what they have done. The past and the present together become the now. With this in mind, many people who have dementia believe that they have already taken a shower. I have clients who will tell me about their typical day, and their spouse will be sitting in my office shaking their head or rolling their eyes. A person with dementia will believe that they are still doing what they did routinely in the past.

2. If someone is not active, they will sweat less. Common sense says that since we are not sweating, why bathe? If a person is no longer doing the activities they once did, such as gardening, cooking, working, or exercising, they may no longer feel that it is necessary to have a daily bath.

3. If we are just going to stay home and no one is going to come over, why bother? Many of us bathe because of social obligations. Even those of us who have no form of memory loss will occasionally have days where we will stay in our pajamas and not wash our face, brush our teeth, or take a bath. Sometimes we just don't care, or we may have other responsibilities that are more important. When I was in graduate school writing papers, I would pick up my daughter wearing the same clothes I wore when I dropped her off. That doesn't sound awful, until I tell you that there were times I stayed in the same clothes for one to two days

depending on the papers I had to write. Because I was so focused on what I was doing, I didn't care how I looked or what I was wearing. The only way I knew that I ate was that my pajama top had stains on it. The difference between my lack of care and a person who is depressed or has dementia is that I was so focused on writing a paper I didn't care how I looked. I had a mother and children to care for and a goal to graduate. Bathing and changing clothes were secondary to my needs. Come Monday morning, when I had to go back into society, I showered, did my hair, and changed into clean clothes. A person who has dementia no longer cares.

4. Many caregivers insist that the person they are caring for has a daily bath. A sponge bath is often a normal bath for those who lived during the Great Depression or World War II or are from different cultures. In earlier times, families would draw one bath that the entire family would use. The elders would bathe first, and then the children would go in, from the oldest to the youngest. By the time the youngest was put into the bath water, it was usually black. This is where the expression "Don't throw the baby out with the bath water" comes from.

5. If a person is depressed, there is no compelling reason for them to bathe. Their thought process is "since life no longer has a purpose, why bother to bathe?" Many of my clients have depression, and because of this, they lose the initiative and desire to bathe.

6. People without memory loss take for granted the steps that are necessary to properly bathe. First,

you have to realize that you need to take a bath or shower. Next, you will have to locate the bathroom. Once in the bathroom, you will have to know how to turn on the shower or bath water, check the water temperature, disrobe, and then enter. Next, you will need to locate the soap and the washcloth or sponge, put the soap on the washcloth, and clean your body by moving the washcloth in the appropriate places. If you need to shampoo your hair, you will have to recognize and then pick up the bottle of shampoo, pour a small amount in the palm of your hand, and then put it on your hair. You must also remember to rinse the shampoo out and then pick up the bottle of conditioner, pour some in your hand, put it on your hair, and rinse it out. Once done, you will need to shut off the shower, locate a towel, and dry off. When a person has dementia, many of these steps may seem impossible or overwhelming. Remember that when a person has memory loss, what was once learned over time will be forgotten. For many, bathing is no longer a pleasurable activity. Bathing is now an anxiety-ridden chore.

7. We take water and swimming in pools or the ocean for granted. In the older days, many people never learned how to swim because they didn't have easy access to lakes, ponds, oceans, or streams. Swimming is a learned experience. Not many people knew how to swim, so many drowned. A lot of people are uncomfortable with water. Daily baths are relatively new. Up until the 1900s in Western culture, baths were taken twice yearly, and additional baths were only taken for special occasions such as births, weddings, and funerals. In

later years, weekly baths became a norm. Families would bathe once a week before going to church or temple. A paycheck on a Friday meant money for coal to heat the water for a bath. Depending on where they lived and the climate conditions, it was not uncommon for people who bathed to suddenly fall ill and then die. There is a generation of people who still believe the old wives' tale that when you bathe, you can catch a chill, become ill, and die. For many people born in the early 1900s and later, water equals illness or drowning. Many of their parents or family members passed the same fear and legacy onto the next generation: those born in the 1910s through the 1940s. These are the persons we are now caring for today.

8. Many of my clients are European survivors of the Holocaust, when over six million Jewish people died. Actually, the numbers rise by the millions when you include many of the innocent people who were murdered who were not Jewish. In the concentration camps, many people were sent to the "showers." People went willingly to the showers because they actually needed and wanted to bathe. A shower represented normalcy, cleansing, rejuvenation, and life. Instead of the anticipated water, human beings were showered with a deadly gas, and they died. If you are caring for a person who lived in Europe during that time, do not use the word "shower." The same rule applies for all members of this generation, no matter whether it is a loved one who was in the Holocaust or a person who has watched the newsreels and press reports about it. Some people who have dementia will become paranoid and aggressive if you ask or tell them that it is time

to take a shower. They may now associate the word "shower" with death. Use the word "bath" or "clean up" instead of shower.

9. Slips and falls in the shower are the number one cause of home injury. I can still remember that each time I announced to my family that I was going upstairs to take a shower, one or both of my parents would say, "Be careful you don't slip." I now automatically say these same words to my kids and continue the bathing paranoia and anxiety.

10. Many women born after the 1920s have a hair ritual. Once a week they either go to a beauty salon where their hair is washed, set, rolled, sculpted, teased, and sprayed or do their hair themselves at home. Once their style is in place, water is the enemy. This is why shower caps and plastic rain bonnets became so popular. It's one more reason why many women will avoid showering. Reassure the person that you will not wet their hair or ruin their "do."

Now you have some additional insight as to why a person may not want to take a bath or shower. Some people, including quite a few doctors, will say that bathing is not a major issue. Many doctors in my area are from foreign countries where their customs of bathing are different. From a social worker point of view, bathing is a major issue. I can only imagine what it would be like to live and sleep with a person who has not bathed in weeks. From what I hear from many of my clients who live with a person who doesn't bathe, it's devastating. Earlier in my practice, my philosophy was "don't sweat the small stuff," and for me, bathing was small stuff. I was naive. When you have a loved one who has not taken a bath for days or weeks, it's big stuff. Some of my clients absolutely refuse to bathe for months at a time and insist that they have recently bathed or have taken a sponge bath. This also happened with my mother, who, while I was growing up, was the cleanest and most well-groomed person I knew. I can remember that as a teenager my mom would beat me by a mile when it came to grooming. I have two teenagers who are the ultimate consumers and groomers. Mom would be proud of her grandchildren's preoccupation with grooming. Once mom had dementia, however, all bets were off. She became King Kong, and it took two aides and me to get her into the shower.

So you may wonder how it comes to the point where a person who once took great care in their appearance suddenly no longer cares or loses interest. First, let me tell you that it doesn't happen overnight. It just seems as if it does. The process has been actually happening slowly, but since you are up close and dealing with a person on a daily basis, it's almost impossible to notice the small subtle daily changes. By sharing close space with another, we adapt to the changes and normalize them. If you have to blame anyone or anything for not noticing the change in the person you care for, blame it on BARK, or beta-adrenergic receptor kinase. BARK controls the functions of the receptors in the brain (and receptors control almost everything that happens in the body). Information from what we see, hear, taste, or touch passes through the thalamus gland for interpretation before it is sent to different parts of the brain and the nervous system. Smell is the only sense that doesn't get processed by the thalamus but is affected by BARK.

The spouse, family member, or caregiver (after spending time with the person) is unaware of a problem because BARK has kicked in. Smell is the most primal of all of our senses. After spending three minutes in any environment, we will adjust to the situation. This is why people who work in restaurants, factories, and trash collection are able to do their job. This is also why parents of babies no longer recognize the smell in their house of their baby's diapers. The same thing applies to people who own dogs or cats. We don't smell our own home, but we can walk into someone else's home and instantly know if they have animals or babies. Our sense of smell is the most primal and developed sense, but in today's world smell is often the most misunderstood, underused, and undervalued of all of our senses. Scent is how newborns in the animal world, including humans, recognize their mothers and how mothers are able to recognize their babies. Our sense of smell triggers memories and emotions.

If a person does not bathe over time, they will have an odor. There is a very small group of people whose sense of smell is so sensitive that BARK never overrides it. A few of these people go on to work in perfume factories or become taste testers. Having a sensitive nose or taste buds can put you into a lucrative field of work. I may have missed my calling to work in the food or perfume industry, but it has been a huge asset to my clients I see in the office or during my home visits. With just one sniff, I know if they have bathed, if they have incontinence, what they ate or drank, and the perfume or even the age of makeup that they wear. When I do a home visit, the way a home smells can tell a lot about the person. Besides incontinence, I can smell mold, the presence of old moth balls, insecticides, and if something in the kitchen has been cooked or burned. My sense of smell is so sensitive it helps me to alert the caregiver to potential situations the caregiver may have overlooked or become accustomed to because of BARK.

We shed our skin daily. Not exactly like a snake that sheds its total skin at one time, but we are constantly shedding pieces of our skin into our clothing, our towels, and our beds. We also shed our skin in the car, on the couch, or on a chair. Anywhere there is friction, you will find dead skin. When we bathe, we remove dead skin by the friction of the washcloth and then drying off with a towel. If we don't bathe, we will continue to remove our dead skin by doing what we do naturally, like tossing and turning in bed. We also remove dead skin by the friction from our clothing when it touches our body. Each movement we make, no matter how slight, will bring us into contact with what we are wearing and help dead skin to shed. Dead skin settles on our clothes, and the bacteria from this layer of skin will cause a "scent" on our clothing. This is why we need to wash an outfit after wearing it. Dust mites live off our shedding skin and for some people can cause allergies (runny or stuffy nose, watery, red, or scratchy eyes).

The same principle applies to bedding. The old saying "Sleep tight; don't let the bed bugs bite" has merit. Bed bugs are real. They feed by sucking blood, and their eggs can be brought into your home by clothes, pets, or furniture. Bed bugs are once again an epidemic. Several high-class hotels have recently been sued because of bed-bug infestation. Bed bugs can cause hives. To reduce the chance of infestation from mites and bed bugs, especially if you are living with a person who is not bathing, you should consider purchasing an encased bed mattress and pillow covers. Wipe down the bed's head board, bottom rails, and foot board. Bed bugs can travel on you and your clothing. Sleeping on the couch might seem like a good option, but if the person hasn't bathed and is wearing the same clothes when they spend time on the couch, chances are the couch is now infested. Some of my clients live in a one-bedroom apartment, so the spouse has nowhere else to sleep—it's either the bed or the couch. If you sleep on the couch, place an open encased mattress cover over the couch before you place your sheets on it. Wash the sheets in hot water daily. If you have a spare bedroom, change into your pajamas in another room before you go into your room. I encourage and recommend separate sleeping arrangements if a person refuses to bathe. Sleeping in the same bed with a person who is no longer bathing is detrimental to your physical as well as emotional health.

So how do you get the person with dementia to bathe? There is no "one size fits all" answer. It will take patience, perseverance, and pressure; pleading and medication can work too. To encourage bathing, here are some suggestions:

1. Determine if the person is depressed. A depressed person, although capable, will not have the needed motivation to bathe. Encourage them to do it, if just for you. If they refuse to bathe, tell them that you have invited friends over for lunch or dinner and that you know that they will want to look good. Or in advance, call up a friend or family member and have them call you at a specific time. When the phone rings, answer it. Walk into the room of the person with dementia and calmly state that the doctor's office called, and they have either moved up the person's appointment or have an opening today. Most people will be motivated to bathe for visitors or doctor's appointments.

2. Check the water temperature. Each of us has what is considered a comfortable level. For me, I will not go into the shower until the water is so hot that you could cook a lobster. Other people might prefer warm or cold. Know their preference before you prepare them to bathe, and set the temperature accordingly.

3. Check the room temperature. We no longer open our windows and let fresh air in; we are now climate controlled. The elderly are especially sensitive to cold air. Anything less than 90 degrees will have many of them putting on sweaters. Their skin is thinner, and they feel the elements more. The thought of having to get undressed and deal with the cold stops many people from bathing.

4. Check the shower pressure. Many shower heads send out water that feels like needles. The elderly have thin and sensitive skin. Replace the shower head with one that sends a softer stream, one that will feel like a gentle rain.

5. People who have dementia are often confused as to what they need to do. Remove the items from the bath area that they do not need or won't be using and have in the shower only the items that need to be used. If possible, purchase a washcloth that you can put the soap in. Pre-measure the shampoo if they are going to wash their hair. Turn the water on, set it to their comfortable temperature level, and then say, "Your bath is ready."

6. Falls are a major concern for the elderly. Many avoid bathing because they are afraid of falling. Install handrails in the shower. If you can (and there is enough space), buy a special bathing seat. Replace the showerhead with a handheld model, so the person who is bathing can control the aim and flow of the water.

7. Shut off the air conditioner, or close off the vents. Shut the windows to increase the temperature in the bedroom for the person to undress. To ensure that

bathing is pleasurable, the bathroom should be a warm and comfortable place.

8. Play music. Music calms the savage beast, and playing music that the person is familiar with and likes may make bath time easier. The person's taste in music will change as the dementia progresses; what works today may not work tomorrow. To be successful, play music that the person grew up with.

9. People with dementia may feel more comfortable and in control if they are given directions. Instead of saying "Would you like a bath?" instead say, "Your bath is now ready."

10. When possible, try to keep to your loved one's past bathing schedule. Some people prefer showering in the morning; some people like to take a shower before they go to sleep. If you keep to their previous bathing schedule, you might have greater success.

11. If the person is having problems with incontinence, they will need to be cleaned. If you can convince them to bathe, you're halfway there. Keep the shower short, let them hold the handheld shower hose, and focus only on the area of their body that needs to be clean. Talk them through what you are doing.

12. Some people are more modest than others. Instead of telling them to take off their clothes, offer them a special towel (Turkish towel) that they can put on before entering the shower that covers their private parts. Once in the shower the person may want to disrobe, but if not, these towels will give them the

comfort they need and you will still be able to help them bathe.

13. Distract the person who is bathing. Place an object in their hand so that they will not fight you in the bathing experience. Have them hold the washcloth, soap, or showerhead, and calmly tell them what you are doing and what they need to do.

14. If a person refuses to bathe, there are products on the market that you can use such as no-rinse soap and shampoo that can simply be rubbed on the body or head. Consider this to be the ultimate in no-fuss bathing.

Above all, keep in mind that a person with memory problems needs to feel safe and secure. If they feel threatened in any way, they will become agitated, anxious, and possibly aggressive. In order to keep things calm, proceed slowly. Reintroduce yourself. Constantly address the person by their familiar name, and tell them who you are. Keep your tone soft, and remain calm. Avoid showing or using anger. Talk them through the steps. If they miss a step or two, do not scold; instead encourage them, and tell them how well they are doing. Once they're out of the shower, praise the person for doing a great job. Offer to help dry them. If the person allows you to dry them, this is a good time to look for body sores, bruises, and abrasions. Unexplained bruises may mean a fall or physical abuse. Suggest putting some moisturizer on them. Many people enjoy some touch. Above all, try to make the bathing experience as enjoyable as possible. If the person still refuses to bathe despite your best efforts, try again later in the day when they may be more receptive. To be successful, it takes trial and error.

Here is my personal trial and error with bathing. When my mother was in the moderate stage of dementia, she absolutely refused to bathe. Just saying the "b" word brought on aggressive behavior. Dad was alive at the time, and he had no success getting her into the shower; my own attempts were beyond pathetic. Nothing I tried worked. So I hired a professional aide, but even she couldn't manage to coax or force Mom into the bathroom (picture a cat that knows that it's going to have a bath). So then I hired two aides to give her a bath. I'm convinced that my neighbors installed impact windows not to keep their homes safe from the hurricanes, but to reduce the sound of my mother's daily screams at bath time. One morning before the two aides came to give Mom her daily bath, she was outside helping me water the plants. I had just had the backyard landscaped, and the new plants needed to be watered with a hose since the sprinklers were not yet installed. As luck would have it, my then three-year-old was riding her bicycle and stopped it on the hose. The water stopped. My mother was confused as to why the water stopped and pointed the hose at herself to see the problem. Just then my daughter got off her bike and lifted it over the hose. Mom got sprayed! (Actually, I refer to that day as the day she got hosed.) I was mortified. I ran to her and apologized and said, "Let's get you out of these wet clothes before you get a chill and get you into a hot bath." Mom went with me willingly to her bathroom, where I ran a hot bath while I got her out of her wet clothes. I helped her with the washcloth and then washed her back for her. God works in mysterious ways. When the aides came later that day, I paid them and sent them away.

The next day, the aides came, and once again it was a battle to bathe Mom. The following day we were out again watering the plants, and this time I purposely stepped on the hose. Once again mom turned the hose from the plants to herself to see what the problem was, and when the hose was aimed at her legs, I stepped off the hose. Once again, her clothes got wet. I ran over to her and said, "Let's get you out of these wet clothes before you get a chill and get you into a hot bath." Again, it worked like magic. This went on for a few months until Mom got over her anxious behavior of not wanting to bathe and, with some prompting and coaxing, could be led into the bathroom.

As caregivers we have so many moments that we get through and then, in time, forget about. The only reason I remembered those moments is that years later I was inside writing a check to the sprinkler guy and something unexpected happened. Picture this moment: Four years later, different house, new landscaping, and Mom is sitting happily outside getting her daily dose of vitamin D with her aide, when suddenly the back sprinklers go on. I'm watching from inside as the sprinklers go on, and my first reaction is horror. Mom's now getting hosed by the sprinklers! Needless to say, the water was quickly shut off. I was angry that my mother's happy day outside was ruined and because of this new situation she might no longer want to go outside. I was freaking out on the inside (forget my conversation with the sprinkler guy) but calm on the outside. Once the sprinklers were shut off, Mom (who was now sopping wet) said to me and her aide, "A hot bath would be nice." God does work in mysterious ways, and despite my fear, Mom's favorite relaxation place for many years was sitting in the backyard.

Dressing

We are what we wear. Society teaches us that the clothes we wear make the person. How we dress sends a message. Who can forget a favorite piece of clothing as a child, the outfit that helped us to feel safe, powerful, and master of our universe? For me, it was a white bathing suit that had black buttons. I was ten years old. I not only slept in it but wore it under my clothes to school. To this day I can still recall the texture and the weave of that bathing suit. This is probably why, when my daughter fell in love with her ballet outfit and wore her tutu everywhere, I never batted an eye. On the other hand, my first born was a totally different matter. I dressed him to the nines. He was color coordinated, preppy, and stylish—an extension of my tastes. Parents flocked to me on the playground. How my son was dressed gave others an indication of who I was and whether I was worthy of being in a specific social circle. Their father had no idea that the way a child was dressed would affect our life. And so there were those few days that his dad would dress Stephen to go to school, when I wanted to put a sign on my child that said, "My father dressed me today." But I didn't, and off he went. However, when I picked Stephen up, I loudly told everyone within earshot that I didn't dress him— his father did! All the mothers laughed and understood.

Looking back on that moment, I know that no matter what age group, people and family members are judged by how a person is dressed. It took me many years living with my son's wardrobe choices to realize that my child's style was not a reflection on me. As a new mother I was looking for acceptance. It took me years, but I finally grew up. I stopped being sensitive to the expectations of others and focused on the needs of my family (which at the end of the day is all that matters). When my daughter went through her phase of wearing a ballerina outfit, her needs came first, and I embraced the moment. When my son (once he became a teenager) went through his Goth phase, I cringed and freaked out for a while, and then I came to realize that he felt comfortable in what he was wearing, and that was what was important. It wasn't about me. It was their stage, their moment, their life. Flash forward to today: my son is the poster boy for Mr. Preppy, and my daughter, little Miss Tutu, will not be caught in public wearing the same outfit twice, unless it's a bathing suit.

Before my mother had dementia, she had more outfits than you can imagine, and for her each day no matter where she was going, she was dressed for a fashion photo shoot. Once Mom reached the moderate stage of dementia, she no longer changed her clothes and would gladly stay in the same outfit day after day. This leads to the importance of understanding dressing and the person with dementia. As caregivers, we may feel that how a person dresses is a reflection of who they are but most importantly who we are. This may be the hardest thing for a caregiver to do, but in order to successfully care for another person; you will need to leave your judgment and self-criticism at the door. This is not about you, nor is it a reflection on you. As this disorder progresses, a person who has dementia will lose interest in what they wear. When a person has any form of memory loss, for some, just the thought of putting on different clothes can be frustrating and overwhelming. Think about the steps involved.

1. Depending on where you are going, you must choose an appropriate outfit.

2. You have to remove the items out of the closet or drawer.

3. The clothes have to be taken off the hanger or unfolded.

4. You will have to put the clothes on in the proper sequence.

5. You will have to figure out how to put the clothes on.

6. Now you must button, zip, or snap the clothes.

7. Next you have to choose the proper belt, tie, scarf, and shoes to go with the outfit.

8. The belt must be pulled through the loops and then buckled or fastened.

9. If you use a tie or scarf, you must secure it correctly.

10. You must put on socks and shoes, in the proper order and on the correct feet.

Whew, I'm exhausted already. Now I know why tennis and jogging outfits are so popular—it's no-stress dressing! But let's review the basic steps of what it takes to be independent:

- plan
- procure
- execute

A person who has dementia will, at different times, have some difficulty being able to choose a particular outfit for their current outing. I have not been diagnosed with dementia, and I have difficulty choosing an outfit. It's a common joke that women whose closets are filled still have nothing to wear. For a person with dementia, dressing is not a joke. It's a debilitating and confusing activity for women and quite a few men. Keep in mind that being properly dressed and looking presentable is important to an individual's sense of self-esteem. If the person with dementia can longer dress themselves properly or be able to choose an appropriate outfit, they will stop attending functions. This can lead to social isolation. As adults, we take dressing for granted. You should keep in mind that surrendering dressing to another person means giving up a part of personal independence: someone else is now choosing for you. Depending on the personality of the person with dementia, some people may easily accept another person choosing their clothes for them. On the other hand, lack of choice or being under the control of another person can cause someone to resist dressing and refuse to cooperate, which may result in aggressive behaviors. The following are some suggestions to make dressing easier.

1. Too many choices will confuse a person with dementia. Pare down the contents of their closet. For some clients, I suggest that caregivers match tops and bottoms for different days of the week. To make choices easier, put a complete outfit together on one hanger, and label each hanger for one day of the week (Sunday, Monday, Tuesday, etc.). Now they have a suitable outfit to wear, which will make their and your life easier. This way they will have a wardrobe that is simplified and easy to manage.

2. Lay their clothing out for them. Place on the bed or a chair every article of clothing that they will need to use. If possible, start from left to right with underwear, socks, shirt, pants, belt, and shoes. Placing items in the order that they need to be put on may help the person with dementia to dress independently.

3. Help them take it one step at a time. The concept of dressing can be overwhelming, and the person who has dementia will be so confused about what to do

that thirty minutes later, when you go back to the bedroom to check on them, you may find them sitting on the bed with a bath towel still wrapped around them. There will come a time when a person who has dementia will need verbal step-by-step commands in order to dress. Encourage them with short, one-step commands. One of my caregivers told me the story of how she told her husband to put his socks on, and fifteen minutes later, when she returned to the bedroom, he still had the pair of socks in his hand. When she asked him why he hadn't put his socks on, he looked at her and said, "I wasn't sure which sock to use— the left or the right one."

4. Choose clothing that is easy to clean. A person with dementia will, at some point, stain their clothes with food or soil themselves. Clothes that need to be dry cleaned should be avoided.

5. If you are purchasing new clothes, buy sweaters that have buttons instead of turtlenecks. At some point, a person with dementia will resist you dressing them, and if you need to pull a sweater over their head, they may no longer be able to understand the concept and will think that they are suffocating. This may cause anxiety and aggressiveness when dressing in the future. Avoid buying pants that need a belt or have buttons or zippers. For the person with memory loss, trying to get their pants off is often the cause of premature incontinence.

6. Walk a person through each step of the dressing process whether they are dressing themselves or you are dressing them. If you are now dressing them, tell

them exactly what it is that you are going to do. If you need to put a shirt over their head, tell them what you are going to do and how they may feel. For example: "This shirt is going to go over your head. For a few seconds, you may feel lost. Don't worry, I'm still here." After you have put the shirt on, praise the person for being cooperative.

7. As we grow older, our bodies shrink in height. Make sure that clothing is not dragging on the floor, which can cause the person to trip or fall. You will also need to be sure that the clothing is not too loose. Giving Mom a bathrobe may seem like a nice gesture, but if the sleeves are too long and could catch on fire while she is cooking, reconsider the gift. Infants' and children's sleep clothing are government-mandated to be flame retardant. Adult clothing is not.

8. Loose clothing is preferable to tight clothing. As we age, our bodies will change. Clothing companies' sizes change, especially for women. A looser bra is a better choice than a tight bra. Clothing that is too tight can cause discomfort, which can lead to a challenging behavior.

9. Foot problems can cause discomfort. Years ago I heard the expression "If your feet are happy, you are happy." It's true. As we age, our foot size will change. In addition, people who have dementia have problems remembering to cut their toenails. Many older individuals develop a toe fungus, which will increase the thickness of the toe, making wearing certain shoes uncomfortable. The longer their toenails, the worse the shoe fit. Recently one of my clients was hospitalized

because of an infection in their big toe that was caused by their shoes. When a person who has dementia is not wearing shoes that are comfortable, they may no longer want to walk, and they may become anxious or aggressive. Sometimes the thickness of the socks may be a problem, or diabetes may be affecting their extremities. Always check the person's feet.

10. Acknowledge special clothes. We all have favorite clothing. There is nothing wrong with wearing the same outfit daily; it just needs to be laundered. If a person with dementia insists on wearing the same clothes repeatedly, try to convince them to put on another outfit, and then have them follow you to the laundry. Wash the clothes they are attached to, and then give them back once they are dry. For some people, certain outfits mean security.

11. Check the person's jewelry. As the dementia progresses, a person may still use clip-on earrings that pinch and cause discomfort. Rings may no longer be comfortable because of swollen fingers. The same goes for watches. As their body changes, you may need to add or take out extra links to make a watch or bracelet more comfortable. Jewelry worn in the daytime, if kept on at night, may become uncomfortable and cause a behavioral disturbance or sleep problems. Heavy necklaces, which are very popular, may make a person with dementia feel they are choking. Each person has a preference. Once when my mother was in rehab, her aide had given her a beautiful pair of clip-on earrings. During a visit I saw my mom tugging at her ears and squirming in her seat. She became agitated and started

grimacing. I took off Mom's earrings, and she instantly calmed down. Who knew that a beautiful gift could cause discomfort?

Eating

Nothing says home like food. Food is a source not only of nourishment but of comfort and socialization. No matter where we were brought up, there are certain foods that will remind us of home and bring us back to our roots—our personal comfort zone. When a person has dementia, food equals love and safety. Food is also a form of medication. For many people with dementia, food holds their memories.

Up until the 1970s, or for some the 1980s, many families shared dinner. Family dinners were a chance for everybody to get together and share their day. Because of lifestyle changes, such as two parents working outside the home and after-school activities, it has become harder for families to keep to a dinner routine. Our elders found comfort in this routine. For many in their generation, it was usual for Mom to stay at home and in the kitchen, while Dad went to work and then came home for dinner. Depending on their culture and preference, some people like to eat early, and others like to eat later. Many people find a sense of comfort, security, and normalcy by staying with or keeping a meal schedule.

For some families, mealtime can be one of the most challenging times of the day, especially if you are caring for a person with dementia. As the course of the disease progresses, the person's eating habits and behaviors may change. Mealtime is not an easy time.

In today's fast-paced world, the concept of dinner has changed. We eat out more often in restaurants, purchase food that is already prepared, and order in more meals than ever before. For many dual-income families or single working parents, meals from scratch are a dream from the past. Mealtime is now just one more chore or responsibility that we need to take care of. You need to keep in mind that, especially for the elderly, mealtime means family and socialization time. Mealtime for them is how they connect or reconnect to the people they care about. Dinner or supper is not always about the meal; it is about being with family and still being a part of a family.

As a person with dementia progresses through the disease, how you adapt and changes that you make will have an effect on not only your life but also theirs. To make mealtime successful, you might need to reevaluate and change your ideal of what a meal is supposed to be.

There can be many causes of eating problems. Some may be from habit, and some are due to changes in the person's brain. Dinner is often the most challenging time of the day because, at this point, most of us are tired after a long day at work or caring for another person. In order to make your family meal successful, here are some suggestions.

1. As the dementia progresses, a person with dementia may have a difficult time sitting quietly at the dinner table. They may become uncomfortable and act out since they are not involved in the conversation, feel left out, or have nothing to do. When you sit down to a meal, in order to avoid a problem behavior, have the meal ready at the table. If this is not possible, provide the person with dementia some finger food that they can manage on their own to keep them occupied.

2. Always check the food's temperature. As the disease progresses, a person with dementia will lose their ability to know if a food is too hot, especially if it is

cooked in a microwave oven. They may burn their tongue or their hand if they touch the food or plate. If you are serving food to a person who has dementia, always check the temperature to be sure that it isn't too hot. On the other hand, if the food is just barely warm or too cold, the person with dementia might not eat it. They will need to have food served to them at their desired temperature.

3. As we age, our senses change. For some people touch, vision, smell, consistency, and taste may diminish. The biggest complaint from elderly who do not have dementia is that food now tastes bland. In order to encourage a person with dementia to eat, you might consider increasing the seasonings. This doesn't mean over seasoning the family meal; just add some additional spices to the food of a person with dementia.

4. Conversations and mealtime for the elderly can be a bad mix. To have a successful meal you will have to balance various factors, including the person's stage of dementia and the generation they were brought up in. My dad was born in the 1890s. The family ate meals together, but no one spoke. Dad's generation was taught that mealtime meant family sitting down together around a table, nobody talking, and each person chewing sixty times for each bite before swallowing, which was suggested by Dr. John H. Kellogg (yes, the cereal mogul) to have good digestion. Dad, who faithfully followed this advice, lived to be ninety-nine years old and remained mentally intact despite his vices. No wonder he was at first appalled and then later amused when as an outgoing young child I would

sit at the dinner table and talk about my day. Imagine his discomfort during our family meals when I was in high school, when the subject would go from the swim team to a class on embalming. All through my life I would bring friends over for dinner. In Dad's time, no one had friends over "because children should eat with their family." Looking back, my college years might have been difficult for my parents because I brought home a variety of opinionated people. As time passed, my father softened and enjoyed my friends and our spirited conversations around the dinner table. Mom enjoyed this time too, until she began to have memory problems, and then dinner time became confusing. She could not keep up with the conversation, had difficulty focusing on what to eat, and often left her plate filled. When you are eating with a person who has dementia, focus on the act of eating. Keep conversation to a minimum. This is not the time to ask questions or to expect answers. A person who is having memory loss will find it difficult, if not impossible, to combine both eating and socializing. Be aware of this, and respect their current limitations.

5. When a person has dementia, you may need to reduce all distractions that can cause confusion, which can lead to anxiety. Some families eat in front of the TV or, even though they are not watching it, keep the TV on as background noise. The same goes for talk radio stations and music. Some of us may find the constant chatter or background noise soothing, but for a person who has dementia, what is normal for us or calms us may cause additional confusion and anxiety. They may no longer understand what is going on while

watching or listening to the nightly news. If anything, hearing about the day's rapes, child abductions, robberies, car accidents, or stock market downturn is no longer a form of entertainment for them. News can be upsetting and unsettling for a person who has dementia. This is because they will at some point lose the ability to separate what is happening on TV or the radio and what is happening in their own life. To have a successful meal, reduce the sound clutter. Turn off the TV and the radio. Avoid spirited conversations. Dad and Dr. Kellogg might have been on to something when they said mealtimes are to eat and chew.

6. Keep food choices to a minimum. Too many choices are confusing for a person who is having problems with their memory. Keep it simple and short (KISS). Ask them what they would like to eat, and offer two choices. This will allow the person with dementia the opportunity to feel good about themselves because they are still able to make a choice. If they refuse to make a choice, try saying, "Mom, would you rather have the chicken or the beef?" or "Mom, since you had steak last night, maybe you would like to have chicken tonight?" If your loved one has difficulty making a decision, it will be up to you to help make a choice. Try saying, "Mom, the chicken looks really good tonight. You order it, and I will order the beef/ fish, and we will share." If possible, order or serve food that the person will like. Common sense says that if a person does not or never has liked a particular food, mentioning or serving it can cause anxiety, not to mention that the person will not eat it! Just because a person has dementia does not mean they no longer

have food preferences. They are still able to know and choose what they like to eat.

7. Try to keep mealtime calm. Keep conversations slow, and avoid confrontations. Mealtime that involves a person with dementia is not the time to deal with your current problems. This is not about you. This is not the time to bring up your difficulties at work, Junior's new tattoo, or the current economic crisis. Topics like these may cause them to have anxiety or agitation, which is why they do not eat or eat less. Resist the urge to vent at mealtime.

8. Encourage a person who has dementia to eat independently. Sometimes you will need to encourage a person who has dementia to eat while still letting them maintain their self-esteem. If you notice that a person is having trouble cutting up their food, do not cut up their food at the table in front of everyone. Instead, cut the food in the kitchen, or have the restaurant worker do it in the kitchen. If the person is having problems using a fork, or spoon, serve them finger foods. Think chicken tenders, steak tidbits, French fries, baby carrots, or other vegetables and fruits that can be easily managed. The goal is to help the person with dementia feel comfortable, confident, and secure at mealtime, and to encourage them to enjoy this time spent together with you and the family.

9. A well-set table, although beautiful, may be confusing for a person with dementia. As their memory disorder progresses, they may have trouble distinguishing the flowers from the salt shakers or recognizing what a fork, knife, or spoon is. As a caregiver, you will need to

simplify the table setting. No matter how pleasing and inviting the table looks to you, it may cause confusion to a person who has memory loss. Remove everything from the table that can or will be a distraction. The two rules of eating are: (1) if it cannot be eaten, do not put it on the table, and (2) if you do not need to use it, do not put it on the table. If Mom is no longer using a knife to cut her food, take the knife away. If the flowers cannot be eaten, take them off the table. If Mom over salts her food, it is due to a reflex action of not being able to stop an action; remove the salt shaker from the table. While you are at it, remove the pepper shaker too.

10. At some point, a person with dementia will have some difficulty eating because they no longer are able to figure out what they need to eat first. If they are having a problem deciding what to eat, they might stop eating altogether. To avoid this situation, try serving one food at a time. On a small plate, place one food in front of the person. For example, start with a plate with a small amount of meat, and after they eat the meat, serve the vegetables, and next place a small amount of potato or rice. Use small portions. Keep in mind that people have food preferences. Some people may not like their food to touch other foods, and others may enjoy eating more than one form of food at a time.

11. Some people might have problems swallowing. I have met many people who have had problems swallowing their food, and they've told me that because of their problem with swallowing, they became self-conscious and avoided eating in front of others. Dementia may cause the food or liquid to go down the wrong "pipe."

Ask your doctor for a swallowing test to determine how best to fix it. Despite what you may think, clear liquids such as water or broth are harder to swallow. You can add certain things to thicken liquids that will reduce swallowing problems, such as a thickening agent prescribed by many doctors (I've tried it and find it unappetizing). An alternative is to add dried mashed potatoes or baby cereal to the food, which will thicken the texture and actually tastes good. If the person likes coffee, try substituting coffee yogurt or coffee ice cream.

12. There may come a point where you will need to adjust the food served or the food's consistency and texture so that a person with dementia will be able to eat, enjoy, swallow, and digest their food. For some this might mean cutting the food up into small pieces; for others it may mean grinding up the meal. No matter what, serve a person with dementia food that is visually pleasing. Ground and pureed food can be shaped to look like the actual food that we normally eat. Serve the food according to the needs of the person. You might need to give them a gentle reminder to swallow between bites.

13. Some people with dementia develop food obsessions. Many of my clients will only eat one type of food and reject others. For some, it may be sweets such as doughnuts or candy; others may crave pasta or ice cream. Carbohydrates are often a favorite. Keep in mind that as the brain is changing, food preferences will change. Try alternating or combining favorite foods with nutritious foods.

14. Some people with dementia overeat. Because of memory loss, many of my clients forgot that they have just eaten. When this happens, simply reduce the size of the meal. Divide the meal in half, and serve it to them at two different times. People with memory loss will not only forget that they ate but insist that they haven't been fed. Instead of arguing or saying that they have just eaten, calmly put the second half of the meal in front of them, and say, "(Breakfast, lunch, or dinner) is served."

15. As the dementia progresses, some people may lose their desire or motivation to eat. For some people, decreased eating is a natural progression of the disease process. Actually, studies have shown that some people who have dementia started to lose weight without trying years before they were first diagnosed. A doctor can prescribe medication to increase their appetite. If you would like to use a behavioral approach instead of or before medication, think red. The color red is a natural appetite stimulant. Think about it: the walls in Italian and Chinese restaurants are often painted red. Many fast food restaurants have the color red in their logo. Most of our homes walls are painted beige or white. In order to increase a person's appetite, add some red. Think about a tablecloth that is red and white. The first thing that pops into my mind is a picnic or barbeque, which means food (yummy) and fun. Actually, it's the food that I think about. To help increase a person's appetite, buy a red tablecloth or a checkerboard cloth, and place it on the table. You can also try red napkins or plastic plates.

As the dementia progresses, food will take on different meanings. It will be up to you, the caregiver, to help the person who has dementia choose the proper food and to help them eat. Over time, the person who has memory loss will have difficulty making decisions. It may appear that they are not interested in eating, but this is not usually the case. It's not that they are no longer interested in food; it is just that there are too many choices to be made or that the whole meal process is too overwhelming. This may be why they avoid going out with family or friends. A person with dementia wants to do what is correct and will avoid making a wrong choice. Faced with a decision that they are no longer able to handle, many may choose not to eat. As a caregiver, the best thing you can do is to give the person with dementia options and then help them choose or direct them. It is also wise to call the restaurant and order the meal in advance, so that when you get there, the meal is ready. It may be a small inconvenience, but it can make for a more successful meal and social outing.

Transferring and Mobility

Transferring is a clinical word for being able to move from point A to point B. It means that you are able to get out of bed, walk to the sofa, and then, when you want, go to the bathroom. Mobility means the ability to move around, which means walking but also includes being able to use a cane, walker, or wheelchair to help you get around. When we were first learning to walk as toddlers, we were a little unsteady on our feet, but with practice, the majority of us eventually managed to make it from the couch to the table. After we mastered it, walking gave us the independence to go places we never could before. Remember the first moon walk: "One small step for man . . ." Walking is the ultimate form of independence!

As adults, if we don't have a physical disability, we often take walking or getting out of a chair for granted until there comes a time in our life when this simple act becomes a difficult or painful experience or downright impossible. Whether it is from normal aging, arthritis, disease, or accident, there may come a time when we need some additional help. Moreover, vision affects memory as well as perception, and if a person is having a vision problem, it will affect their ability to walk by themselves, which will affect their independence. An inner ear problem can affect balance. Having difficulty walking will affect socialization, toileting, bathing, feeding, dressing, and behavior.

Keep in mind that any person who is having memory loss is going to have difficulty walking. Walking is a learned behavior, and any behavior that is learned will at some point be forgotten. Let's look at some of the ways that walking difficulties and transferring will affect the person who has dementia.

1. Most of us get pleasure from being with other people, and socializing is for many people a major pleasure in their lives. People who have dementia may be more prone to falling or feel uncomfortable leaving the safety of their home. Many of my clients are embarrassed to be seen outside of their home with a cane, walker, or wheelchair, and because they need additional assistance, they start to socially withdraw. Out of pride, many people with dementia who have problems with walking would rather stay home than go out in public. This holds true for those people who have no cognitive problems. Most people avoid using a cane or walker because they think that it makes them seem old, feeble, and dependent.

2. If a person is having mobility problems, they may have problems getting to the bathroom. Many of my clients are not incontinent in the true sense of the word; they are just having problems making it to the bathroom in time. Because of their slow walking or because they might need the aid of another person to help them out of the bed or chair (transferring), accidents happen. This can cause embarrassment and isolation.

3. The distance to the bathroom to bathe, although just a short distance, may seem like a journey of a hundred miles to a person with dementia. Trying to support themselves on unsteady legs in the shower is scary. If a person is having trouble getting out of a chair, the thought of needing help getting out of a bathtub is worse. Many people with dementia will refuse to bathe because of their problem with mobility.

4. Many of my clients' eating problems are caused by their lack of mobility. They are used to eating in restaurants, but having to navigate a restaurant with a cane, walker, or wheelchair can be a daunting and difficult experience. If someone can no longer drive or walk to their favorite restaurant, they stay home. Ordering in or having meals delivered is not familiar for some people. Dinner at the home of a family member or friend can cause anxiety. Once seated in the living room, a person with dementia will have to get up off the sofa and walk to the dining room, locate where they are to be seated, and then sit down. This can cause self-consciousness and be difficult to manage. Preparing a home-cooked meal means standing on your feet in the kitchen, something people with dementia may no longer be able to do. If a person

is having problems with mobility or transferring, they may go without eating.

5. Dressing takes energy and stamina. Going to the closet and then choosing and putting on clothes is a hard task. Standing to choose the clothes and put them on takes time and energy. For my clients who have trouble walking, the thought of dressing sends them back into their bed. Standing is difficult; getting off the bed is difficult. For the person who has mobility problems, it's easier for them to lie in bed in their pajamas, and just stay home.

As a caregiver you need to be aware that mobility and transferring problems may cause additional behaviors such as isolation, anxiety, or aggressiveness. They may now exhibit anger because they have lost some of their independence, and most likely they will take out their frustration on you. On the other hand, a person may become more docile. Since they can no longer walk by themselves or move from point A to point B without the help of another person, they may resign themselves to the fact that they will need help, or they may refuse to move at all. As a caregiver you will need to help this person through motivation or physical aids to keep them active and engaged.

ADLs and IADLs mean independence. Think back to a time when you needed to depend on others to get through the day. Over the years I've broken limbs, been sick, had surgeries—I'm surprised that my family tolerated me! It's not that I didn't appreciate their help. I was just frustrated that I needed their help! I'm not good when it comes to accepting care and being dependent on others, even when I know that it's temporary. The same thing goes for a person who is having memory loss. For many people who have dementia, especially in the early stages, they may experience moments of sadness. The life they are leading is not the life they had envisioned. They are grieving over a loss, and this is often misdiagnosed as depression. We all want to remain independent, but sometimes life throws us a curveball. As a caregiver, you will need to be the cheerleader. Remember that no matter who you are dealing with, they are still a human being who deserves respect.

CHAPTER EIGHT

DEALING WITH UNWANTED BEHAVIORS

A behavior will be unwanted for three reasons: it is new to you, you have never experienced it before with this person, or it is causing a disruption in your life. You are used to dealing with your loved one based on past experiences; now you have a new relationship. Any new relationship will take time to adjust to. This is especially true when dealing with a person who has dementia. Despite all of the years you have known this person, you are dealing with a different individual. They may look the same on the outside and sound the same, but their brain is changing inside. As a caregiver, you are not going crazy or imagining things. The reality is that any person who has dementia will go through a period or periods of time when their confusion and disorientation will cause a behavior or personality change.

Some of these periods last for a few seconds; some last for minutes, hours, or days; others may last for months. Rarely will they last for years. The most difficult part of your job as a caregiver will be learning how to manage an unwanted behavior while keeping some normalcy in your life. The next five words, if you take them to heart, will change the way you view and deal with a challenging behavior: *Every behavior has a reason.*

In chapter 4, you learned that there are pharmacological ways to deal with challenging behaviors. Remember that many medications are developed for and tested on persons younger than sixty-five years old. Many of the drugs prescribed to calm or stop a behavior are most commonly used on younger individuals who have depression, schizophrenia, anxiety, or sleeping disorders. Medication may help in the short term, but it may also have short- and long-term side effects. Often people with dementia are on several medications simultaneously for health or behavioral reasons. Medication side effects can be the cause of the current and unwanted challenging behavior.

I am not anti-medication, but I am opposed to overuse of medication. If a medication can stop an unwanted or challenging behavior and gives you back your life and the person with dementia returns to some kind of normal state, then I am all for it. For many caregivers who are under stress or misinformed, medication is often their first line of defense. But in fact environmental and behavioral changes, while they may take a little longer, often get the same result as medication without the side effects.

This chapter will help you gain a better understanding of some of the most common behaviors that a person with dementia might have. Remember, your journey is unique, and the person you are caring for is one of a kind. Because you know your loved one so well, any change in their current behavioral pattern is going to be confusing, exasperating, and annoying, or on the opposite side, you may accept the change or never address it. I will help you understand what is going on in the mind of the person with dementia and give you the tools to deal with the current situation.

As a result of the changes in their brain, the person with dementia will begin to have difficulty with language, judgment, reasoning, sequencing, and planning. They may also have difficulty with perception and motor skills. All of this combined will result in their inability to carry out their normal daily activities. These are the things that you and I typically take for granted—like taking a bath, brushing teeth, taking medication, planning a dinner, etc. Some professionals in the field of dementia use a timeline that predicts when certain behaviors might occur, but I no longer use one. After many years in the field, after observing my mother and clients at day centers and speaking with thousands of clients and colleagues, I have learned that each person is unique and that behavioral problems may start earlier or later in some people. For some, behavioral problems never occur. It all depends on the person, the kind of memory loss they have, their environment, their personality, and their caregiver.

For many people with dementia, the first sign of the illness is a change in the individual's personality. If the person is having memory loss, any change in their brain is a change that you or they cannot control. No matter how valid your points or observations are, you will not be able to reason with a person who has dementia. They are changing, and they are no longer capable of making certain decisions or controlling their actions or responses. Who they are and where they are right now dictates how you'll need to adjust and adapt to their moment. I say "their moment" because when dealing with a person who has dementia, it is all about them. A person with dementia is in the emotional driver seat, and as a caregiver you are now in the back seat. By the time you are done reading this book you will be a great back-seat driver.

Every behavior has a reason behind it. A person with dementia is just trying to survive—to look for the familiar. The familiar may be a time or place where they feel (or felt) safe. To get through this day or moment, a person with dementia will use whatever resources they currently have available as well as their memories of what worked for them in the past.

When a person has any form of dementia, over a period of time they will lose their ability to communicate their needs, wants, and desires. They will eventually lose the ability to figure out what it is that they want to tell you, and they will lose the ability to describe what it is that they desire or need. Keep in mind that you are now dealing with a person who is desperately, and in their own way, trying to hold on to their current lifestyle and independence—the familiar. The person with dementia is not concerned with you; they are concerned and consumed with themselves. What you see as an unwanted or challenging behavior has a purpose for the person who has memory loss. Survival and control are important for them. Behavioral problems are responses that allow the person with memory loss to use the coping skills that they once used successfully to get through the moment.

A person with dementia will have difficulty with language, judgment, reasoning, sequencing, and planning. Because of this they will forget how to act or what to do. As a caregiver, you have a tough road in front of you. Managing a challenging behavior is going to be one of the most difficult tasks that you will have to face as a caregiver. To be a successful caregiver, part of your job is to help the person with a behavioral problem get through their moments, to understand what these moments represent to the person, and, at the same time, to retain your sanity and—hopefully—your sense of humor. This is not a job for the meek. Remember: no matter how difficult or challenging the behavior is, it will eventually stop on its own.

Lesson One: *Letting Go of Familiar Behaviors*

With dementia, familiar behaviors now may be causing frustration, miscommunication, fear, anxiety, or anger for the person with dementia or the caregiver or both. For a couple who has been married for years and whose form of love and communication was to bicker, when the person with dementia no longer can bicker, they become anxious, agitated, or physically and/or verbally abusive toward their spouse. This situation can cause resentment or anger for both parties. I also see clients who had relationships in which they used "love taps" or pinching to show affection or displeasure. The person with dementia no longer responds to these actions and instead feels threatened and will strike back, either physically or verbally, with a vengeance. Out of frustration, some people with dementia will strike their spouse or caregiver. Out of frustration, some caregivers will strike the person in their care.

Always keep in mind that the person who has dementia has a brain that is not only changed but constantly changing. They might not always remember or be capable of responding in their former ways. If you playfully hit them, they might not remember that this is a part of the relationship; they may hit you back really hard. To successfully deal with a person who has dementia, you will need to develop a new approach for successful communication. This will not be easy. It is hard to break familiar habits and patterns, but it will be necessary if you want to help the person with dementia and yourself.

Why is letting go of old familiar behaviors so important? Because the person with dementia will have brain changes that they have no control over. How they act or react is no longer in their control. Many of their responses are now primal: they need to be understood and survive. As a caregiver, you can control what you do. You have the capacity to see what is happening and, most importantly, change the way that you respond to the person with dementia. Unlike the person with dementia, who has lost their ability to reason, you have the ability to make choices and to change your communication style and behaviors if they are no longer working for either of you.

Each day, a person who has dementia will go through several behavioral stages. At times, they may be independent or needy, remember or forget, or be capable or incapable. There is no rhyme or reason to this disorder, and it will affect each person differently. As a caregiver, you need to shift your perspective of your loved one. You want them to be their "familiar" normal self so that you can continue in your previous comfortable existence. The idea that they are no longer the person you know may cause you to overreact. Caregivers can have a tendency to go to extremes too! They will either push a person further than they are capable of or protect and baby them. A caregiver will often discount the abilities of the person with dementia based on the caregiver's own needs.

We allow a person with memory loss to continue to drive their car when they really shouldn't because we want them to be independent, or because we need them to drive since we can't, or because we cannot be there for them. We allow the person with dementia to handle the family finances even when we know they are having problems balancing the checkbook, paying bills, or dealing with the stock broker or accountant, because we are clueless when it comes to finances or do not have the time to get involved. We allow the person with dementia to cook even when we know that they are no longer able to use the stove or be safe with sharp knives because they have always been the cook in the household. Often a person with dementia will insist or demand that they are capable of doing things they no longer can in order to remain independent. As caregivers, we often give in and support a person's independence even when we know that the person is no longer capable of doing things safely or living independently. The reason we do so is to keep our life normal and to avoid a confrontation.

Sometimes we let a person with dementia to continue to rule the family because we need them to be the head of the family. For some of us, this may stem from a religious or cultural upbringing. Our culture and family of origin play a role. The television shows we grew up with also play a role. We have been taught to respect our elders, but nobody has taught us what to do when our elders are no longer capable of taking care of themselves. Often the dad was the head of the household. For years you may have heard, "This is your father's decision, and what he say goes." In the past, Mom controlled the house by day and, in order to back herself up, would say those infamous words that sent shivers down our spines, "Wait until your father comes home." In other families it was Mom who had control or another family member, but the result is the same. We do not want to assume responsibility out of fear of offending them, fear of change, or because we're in denial.

Many families are downright scared of offending the person with dementia and will, because of their fear, allow the person to maintain control. Once you come to grips with the fact that a person with memory loss is having a problem, it will be up to you to take control of the situation. Ignoring the situation will not make it go away; over time it will only get worse. Role reversal, for some family members, may be strange and hard at first, but it's something that you will have to do if you want to successfully care for a person with dementia. It's not going to be easy, and it will take time and guidance to help you get through it. There are some family members who have always been controlling, and due to their memory loss they are now unreasonable. Just like when it comes to adding any new medication, you will need to start low with small changes and go slow. Depending on you and your family's situation, taking control may mean being personally involved with daily care, hiring someone to help, finances, medical care, or a mixture of all.

Lesson Two: *Common Behaviors for People with Dementia*

When you are dealing with a person who has dementia, you have to keep in mind that their current behavior is influenced by their past behavior. A person with dementia is looking for the familiar. They are now using their past coping methods to deal with the current situation. Depending on your relationship with this person, how you approach the person with dementia will put you in their mind as either a helper or an intruder. The level of help you offer and (here is the key point) the amount of help they accept will depend on their current mental state, your relationship with them (real or imagined), how they view you, and your understanding of this disorder.

Challenging behaviors can be placed into two different categories: emotional and physical. What a person with dementia feels and believes affects their emotional and physical state, which you as a caregiver will now be dealing with.

The following lists should *not* be used as a guide to what will happen to the person you are caring for; these are only potential emotional states and behaviors of a person with dementia. Just because your loved one does one thing does not mean that they will experience all of the things in these lists. I have many clients with dementia who have done few if any of these things. I also have some clients who have experienced all of these things on these lists—and more.

Common emotional states and emotional behaviors include:

- anxiety
- depression
- hallucinations
- combativeness
- screaming, cursing
- hostility
- paranoid thoughts
- hitting, kicking, biting, or throwing things
- overreacting to a situation
- delusions
- mood swings
- being tired
- lack of interest

Common physical behaviors include:

- wandering
- pacing
- stealing someone's property
- shadowing (where they follow you around)
- repetitive speech and/or actions
- restlessness
- inappropriate toileting
- undressing
- sexual hyperactivity
- feeding problems
- sleeping problems
- sundowning*
- rummaging (repetitive nonproductive activities such as opening and closing a purse or drawers)

* Sundown syndrome is the result of disorientation that occurs as daylight decreases, in the early to late afternoon and evening; a person who is sundowning may get anxious, aggressive, or paranoid. There will be more on sundown syndrome later in this chapter.

Lesson Three: *Understanding Behavior Changes*

For just one moment, I would like for you to imagine what it would be like if you woke up one morning different from the person you were when you went to sleep. You've changed, but nobody realizes that you've changed because you still look the same, only with minor differences that are unnoticeable to anyone but you. The family treats you the same and expects you to react the same. It is a Kafkaesque moment. I'm referring to the short story "The Metamorphosis" by Franz Kafka, written in 1915. It is the story of Gregor Samsa, who went to sleep and awoke the next day recalling the strange dream he had where he lost his personhood and was transformed into a bug. Overnight, Gregor slowly became a bug. Actually, he became a cockroach. He knew he was now a bug, but nobody in the family recognized or acknowledged his change. The family kept their life normal by acting as if Gregor were normal. The more they pretended that Gregor was normal, the larger he grew as an insect. As a family, they never accepted the changes that Gregor was going through and denied the situation. The family went on as usual, ignored Gregor's changes, and pretended that Gregor was still the person they knew him to be. It's not outrageous to suppose that Kafka himself might have had a family member or friend with dementia.

As a caregiver you need to keep reminding yourself that any change in behavior or any unwanted behavior is not purposefully done to annoy you, guilt-trip you, or manipulate you. A person who has dementia, because of the changes in their brain, is as powerless as you are to stop their behaviors. Their brain is changing- it is shrinking and filling up with gunk—plaques and tangles. Any change that happens in the brain will have an effect on how a person thinks, acts, or responds. No matter what happens, always remember that if the person's brain was functionally normal, they would not be engaging in these new behaviors that are now foreign, confusing, and confounding to both of you.

When dealing with a disruptive behavior, keep in mind that decades of personal conflict that have been repressed may be now coming to the surface. You should also realize that a person who is having memory problems will fight to avoid danger. For them, danger is the unknown. Anything out of the ordinary is now considered to be dangerous. Since the person is now having difficulty with processing information, they may perceive many things—including their own thoughts— as a threat. Disruptive behaviors are a survival reaction and an attempt to return to the familiar.

As the disorder progresses, their actions will seem unreasonable to you. As caregivers, we too may become unreasonable. In our own minds, we think that we are acting rationally. Imagine how you feel when another person tries to stop you from doing what you want to do, or what you think it is that you need to do. In this situation you will become defensive, and your personal survival reaction to react kicks in. It's just human nature. Often it's not the other person's behavior that causes so much trouble; it's our behavior—the behavior and mind-set that we have locked ourselves into. Believing that our way is the right way, or the only way to do thing, limits our options. Each of us has our own comfortable way that works for us (or we think that it does) to deal with problems or relationships. Once we are out of our comfort zone, we will act or react differently. People affect our comfort zone as well as our environments.

When you are dealing with an unwanted behavior from a person who has dementia, first determine what it is you want to happen. Ask yourself the following questions:

1. What do I want them to do or expect them to do differently?

2. Am I being reasonable?

3. Is my reaction valid?

4. Is the problem real or an annoyance?

5. Does the behavior pose a safety risk to the person with dementia or to me?

You will need to keep in mind that a person who is having a memory problem has a progressive irreversible brain disorder. This will make it difficult for them to:

- Learn new tasks and remember the steps that we naturally take for granted.

- Process complex information.

- Rely on their perceptions and be able to communicate.

- Understand their environment.

To successfully deal with a person who has dementia, you will have to start where the person is today. It's no longer about you. It's now all about them, just like dealing with a toddler or teenager—or a boxer in a different weight class. The person's personality and their level of dementia will affect how they are able to handle the current situation. You will need to work within their reality; you will not be able to change their reality. There is nothing you can say or do that will change how they think or why they think what they do. To be a successful caregiver, you will have to be able to find a way to follow their current train of thought, validate their concerns, and, if necessary, use a distraction technique.

Lesson Four: *Determining the Cause of an Unwanted Behavior*

Before you start any behavioral intervention, you should first rule out any medical problem that can be the cause of this new behavior. A sudden or new change in behavior can be a result of a physiological change that may be treatable such as a urinary tract infection or even the common cold. People with dementia are at a greater risk of having a compromised immune system, which makes them more vulnerable to infections. Many of these individuals have additional concerns such as diabetes, blood pressure, and heart problems. A new medication may cause a behavioral change. They may also be in physical pain. When it comes to a new disruptive behavior you need to ask these questions:

- Could this new behavior be due to a medication reaction?
- Is there an acute illness?
- Is there a chronic illness?
- Is the person dehydrated?
- Is the person constipated?
- Could they have an infection?
- Are they in physical discomfort?

If you are not sure what is causing a new behavior, call their primary care doctor. If you are unable to reach them because it is a very busy office or it is after hours, call 911.

If you feel that the situation is life threatening, immediately call 911. It is not uncommon for a person who has dementia to suddenly develop an infection, and a new behavior may be their only sign of alerting you that they are having a problem. Do not second-guess this situation. It's better for you to be embarrassed by a false alarm than to find out later that your loved one's distress was a true medical condition.

If a person is having a disruptive behavior and you have ruled out a medical condition, the next step is to explore the current environment as a factor for this new behavior. For some people, the environment they are living in may cause confusion. As the person's memory loss progresses, their orientation will change. As they age, their vision and hearing change, as well as their sense of touch and smell. This will add to sensory deprivation and add to the stress and confusion to the person who is having memory loss. Their changes in perception and in communication ability will mean what was once familiar for a person with dementia will now be an obstacle. Ask yourself these questions:

- Could their environment now be confusing?
- Does the person with memory loss have sufficient orientation?
- Check the sensory environment. How is the lighting? Is there glare? Does the floor pattern allow for comfort and maneuverability?
- Is the environment unstructured?
- Is the home cluttered?
- Is there too much or too little stimulation?
- Is the temperature too cold or too hot?
- Are the bathroom and bedroom clearly marked?

The next thing you should look at is capability. A person may look the same on the outside, but you will need to recognize and accept that they may no longer be the same independent person you once knew. Over time they will lose some of their abilities to do what they once did with ease. Mom may no longer be able to pull together the Thanksgiving dinner by herself, or Dad may now have difficulty being the family's financial consultant or handyman. As a caregiver and as an adult, you will need to accept and work though these changes. This won't be easy. If you have always depended on your spouse to provide you with emotional or financial support, this may be really hard for you to handle. In order to help the person who is having memory loss, you will have to realize that some tasks are now beyond your loved one's current capabilities. It may be helpful to remember the following:

- As the brain changes, a person's perception of the situation will change.

- Their lack of communication skills will make it hard for the person with dementia to understand what is expected from them.

- Because of their communication problem, it may be difficult for you to understand their current wants and needs.

As a caregiver, you have wants, needs, and expectations of the person you are caring for. It can be hard to accept that the person you love has changed, because they may look the same and have "normal" moments, and so you will grab onto these fleeting moments and push aside your fears and doubts of what is happening. The reality is that at times it will not be easy and will be downright scary: a future of the unknown seems worse than taking control of the now. And taking control of the now as a caregiver is what you will need to do no matter how uncomfortable it may be to you.

Lesson Five: *Understanding Environmental Stressors*

An environmental stressor is anything that will cause a person with dementia to no longer feel comfortable. "Comfortable" is another word for safe. A person who has memory loss wants to feel safe, to be in their familiar. If they don't feel safe, they may act out. The acting out is actually a self-soothing process to gain a feeling of safety. At this point, they are unaware of what they are doing or how it affects you. Acting out is a way to regain a sense of their safety and allows them to be in familiar territory. For a person with dementia, safety and comfort are their number one priorities. At this point, you are no longer a thought in their mind. Their goal is to be safe, feel safe, and maintain a sense of self and dignity. Anything that challenges their sense of safety, self, or dignity will cause a behavioral disturbance. The following is a short list of potential environmental stressors:

1. New surroundings. For a person with dementia a new surrounding can mean any number of things. It can be a change in where they live, a visit from a family member, having a family member come to live with them, or temporarily being in a new environment—like going to a restaurant or the mall or even visiting a doctor's office. People who have memory loss feel safe in their familiar routine. A change in their routine will be upsetting to them. Remember, there will come a time when every moment is a new moment for them.

2. Fabric patterns. Some people are color or pattern sensitive. If they are in a room that has loud, brash, or

confusing colors on the walls or furniture, they may get agitated. The same goes for patterns. Many homes have a black-and-white pattern on the wallpaper or floors that was once popular in the 1960s and 1970s, which now can be visually confusing.

3. Lack of routine. You may think that doing the same thing over and over again would be boring. It might be for you, but for the person with dementia a routine is very comforting. They know what is going to happen and can plan accordingly. Just like a young child who watches the same movie or reads the same book over and over again because it is familiar and they know what to expect, a person who has dementia feels secure when they have a routine.

4. Stimulation. There is a fine balance between overstimulation and under stimulation. A comfortable degree of activity will vary depending on the time of day and the person. Too much stimulation can cause agitation and aggressiveness. Too little stimulation can cause boredom, isolation, social withdrawal, agitation, or depression.

5. Lack of orientation. Not being able to recognize friends or family members, locate the bathroom or familiar places, or determine what utensil to use at the dinner table can cause stress.

6. Lighting. As we age, our vision changes. What is comfortable lighting to you can cause a person who has memory loss to experience disorientation, hallucinations, delusions, or sundowning and can add to depression. In short, improper lighting can cause many unwanted behaviors. Depending on the time

of day and the surface, sunlight may cause temporary blindness, and the person may refuse to go outside.

7. Noise. Loud or unwanted noises can increase agitation in the person who has dementia. People with dementia are very sensitive to sound, and since many of them have difficulty understanding where the sound comes from, anything that is loud or abrasive will assault their sense of comfort. A person who has dementia will have difficulty understanding noise. Noise is stimulation. Conversation is stimulation. For the person who has dementia, sitting at the dinner table where two to three conversations are going on at once may be stimulation overload. Listening to music that they do not like or that is in a foreign language can cause anxiety. Actually, listening to any music you do not like is a form of torture. The constant whining of a grandchild may cause an unwanted behavior, and so can the barking of a dog, meowing of a cat, or sound of a neighbor's lawn mower.

8. Room temperature. We all have a personal temperature comfort zone. When it comes to behaviors, temperature is important. A person who has dementia is very sensitive to temperature. If the temperature in the room is too high or too low, it may cause agitation, sleep disorders, or other unwanted behavior.

9. Flooring. Since this is where we walk, the floor is a form of security. For a person with dementia, a shiny waxed floor is no longer just a clean floor—it is an obstacle. Shiny equals water; water means slip; slip means fall; fall means nursing home; nursing home means death. This is the thought process of a person

with moderate and severe dementia. Contrasting floor colors may cause a person with dementia to change their walking behavior. Dark colors mean holes. Holes mean a fall, a fall translates to being in a nursing home, and a nursing home means death. This may be why someone with dementia would rather stay on the couch or in their bed.

10. Mirrors. There will come a time when a person with dementia forgets what they look like. When they look in a mirror or see their reflection in a window at home, in a store, or in the car, they think a stranger is watching or following them. Mirrors, television, or a family portrait may bring on what we might think of as a delusion or hallucination.

11. Clutter. A person with dementia will need clear spaces to feel comfortable and be able to walk around. A person with dementia will eventually have a problem understanding the concept of furniture, pictures, magazines, and even television. In chapter 9 ("Home Safety"), I will deal with these issues in more depth.

Lesson Six: *Understanding Physical Stressors*

Other stressors can be due to physical problems. A person with dementia will at some point lose their ability to explain what makes them feel uncomfortable. Because of their lack of communication ability, you'll need to be sensitive to possible clues. You will need to put yourself in the shoes of the person who has dementia and try to figure out what is making them uncomfortable. Once again, if a person with dementia is having a new or difficult behavior, the first thing you should always rule out is an infection. Any behavior that appears suddenly and is out of their normal range needs immediate medical intervention. The following is a short list of possible physiological stressors.

1. Clothing. As we age, our body naturally changes. We get wider and shorter. We still want to believe that we will always fit in the same size clothes. Family members often buy clothes that are ill-fitting, usually too loose or too tight. Loose clothes can be a safety hazard if the clothes cause tripping while walking, catch on an object, or have sleeves that can catch fire while the person is cooking. Wearing clothes that are too tight is uncomfortable and constricting, which can contribute to behavior problems. When evaluating your loved one's clothes, consider all items: socks, underwear, bras, shirts, pants, skirts, shoes, socks, suspenders, and even jewelry. As the dementia progresses, the person with memory loss may no longer be able to tell you what is uncomfortable for them, so they will act out.

2. Foot problems. People with dementia will have corns and calluses that will need to be addressed. They may also have a toenail fungus, causing one toenail, usually the big toenail, to become so thick that it makes wearing closed-toe shoes uncomfortable. Shoes that fit well in the morning may be uncomfortable later on in the day. Having a pedicure is nice, but a monthly visit to a podiatrist is a must.

3. Mouth problems. A person with dementia can develop problems with their teeth that can cause them discomfort. As people age, their mouth space changes, and so does bone density, which will affect their mouth structure. Dentures that once fit well now no

longer do. The person with dementia will not be able to brush and floss the way they once did. If a person has a toothache, they may lose their appetite or have behavior problems. Keep the twice yearly visits while the person with dementia is still capable of sitting in a dentist chair. As the dementia progresses, there may come a time when your loved one will need to be medicated to have any dental work done. Check with their neurologist before any medication is given.

4. Vision problems. Light is a main source of behavioral problems. People over sixty years old need more light, and, at the same time, this light can sometimes be overwhelming. Light affects a person's perception of things and can have an effect on behavior. Over time, dementia will cause visual spatial problems, and a person will misjudge objects and distance. They may no longer be able to copy or trace a simple diagram on paper. What they actually see and the object being seen are for them two different things. As a caregiver, you might think that a person is hallucinating—for example, if they believe that the coat rack in the hallway is a man with a hat.

5. Wounds. No matter whether the person with dementia is recovering from surgery or has some type of injury, they are going to be uncomfortable. Each of us has a different level of pain tolerance. Memory loss makes it difficult to describe the pain or where the pain is located. Many people with dementia cannot recall what happened to them. I have had clients who have fallen out of bed and will get back up and return to bed. Because they found a way back into their bed, the caregivers didn't know that they fell. After watching

the person's body language and listening to the sound of their voice, I recognize that something is wrong. Often times they are in pain. In this case I advise the family to call the primary care doctor, who usually will order an x-ray. Nine times out of ten, the pain was caused by a broken bone or a fracture. If a person with dementia starts to hold a body part such as a shoulder, arm, or leg, they may have an injury. Request an x-ray or an MRI. It's better to be safe than sorry.

6. Bruises. Some bruises cause pain. A person with dementia will forget how they got the bruise and will not be able to tell you. They may have gotten burned by the stove while they were cooking, or they may have fallen or accidentally bumped into another object. Bruising may mean an infection or a broken bone.

7. Abuse. A bruise may also mean that a person might be abused. If a person has unexplained bruises that are not the result of a fall or in an area of their body that can't be easily explained, there is a possibility that the person might be abused. Because of their lack of communication skills a person with dementia is vulnerable and an easy target for physical or verbal abuse.

8. Prescribed medication. Mismanagement of medication may cause unwanted behaviors. Many of my clients overmedicate or under medicate themselves. They may forget that they already took a dose and then will take it again, or they may not believe in medication and will either reduce the dose that was prescribed or not take it at all. Some well-meaning caregivers who have

their own beliefs about medication will adjust the dosage without consulting first with the doctor.

9. Medical conditions. Shingles or herpes may cause extreme pain that will be hard to explain. Arthritis will cause pain and so will back and hip problems. Sinus problems and headaches can cause additional pain.

As a caregiver you need to keep in mind that a person who has dementia may also have physical, medical, and emotional problems that will have to be understood and addressed.

Lesson Seven: *Understanding Anxiety*

When a person is anxious, they are nervous, tense, agitated, and unable to focus or concentrate. Anxiety is an internal response to an inner stress that grows into an external reaction. The external reaction results in a behavior. When a person is anxious they will worry about anything and everything. An anxious person will have problems sleeping because their brain is constantly racing. The fear of knowing they have something important to remember but forgot what it was often causes them to be repetitive. They may ask the same question over and over again. They may also open and close their purse, sort and repack clothing, constantly check that the door is locked, or pace from room to room. The person is in continuous motion that seems to lead nowhere. It's like living with the Energizer bunny; they just keep going and going and going. The commercials are amusing and entertaining, but living with a person whose behaviors keeps going and going is difficult. Some of the behaviors an anxious person may engage in is pacing, fidgeting, and being verbally or physically repetitive. Some of these behaviors are self-soothing for the person with dementia. Their constant smoothing of their clothes may drive you nuts, but for the person with dementia, this action is calming.

A person who is anxious is insecure. They will need reassurance from you that all is well. To successfully deal with a person who is anxious, you will need to assure and reassure them that they are safe. If they are looking for a lost item, offer to help find it. If they are concerned about their finances, talk with them, and show them (if needed) a recent bank or brokerage statement. No matter what, do not argue with them (you will never win). Be consistent in your answer and response. Above all, remain calm. If the situation gets tense or increases, distraction may be your best defense. Many times, distracting the person with a change of scenery or with food may help to calm the person. When you are dealing with a person who has anxiety, the best course of action is to keep them within a familiar routine. This is not the best time to go on an outing, have friends over, go to a restaurant, or walk the mall. When a person is anxious, something as simple as walking in an unfamiliar direction can lead to increased panic, confusion, and anxiety.

Here are some behavioral management techniques that have been successful in coping with anxiety:

1. Use a calm voice. Tone is important; this will set the stage for what you need to do.

2. Use touch. A smile, hug, or calming hand can work wonders.

3. Place visual clues to give structure. Mealtimes are important. Make or buy a clock that shows the time that breakfast, lunch, and diner will be served.

4. If a person can no longer read, use symbols. Tape a picture of the toilet on the door of the bathroom. Make signs for the kitchen and bedroom.

5. Don't discuss a future event. Any event out of the "now" moment is a future event. If you tell a person with dementia that tomorrow they have a doctor's appointment, they may ask questions repeatedly, become agitated or aggressive, or lose sleep. Instead, say nothing. Try to keep things as normal as possible. When the person is dressed and you are ready to leave, calmly say, "We are going out now." If they ask where, tell them that you are both going to visit the doctor. If you know that going to a doctor's appointment will cause them anxiety, don't say where you are going; instead say, "It's a surprise." Have something fun planned before or after the appointment such as eating lunch out or going to an ice cream parlor. I call this "a loving deception." There is no reason to cause additional anxiety to a person who has dementia.

6. Listen to the emotion in their voice and note their body language instead of asking specific questions. Sometimes a person is just looking for reassurance that everything is going to be okay. Reassure them that all is well.

7. Keep your answers brief and simple. Remember, many people with dementia will lose track of a sentence after the third word. Complex explanations will cause confusion, which will lead to an increase in anxiety and agitation.

8. A person who has dementia does not realize that they have asked the same question once, twice, or what

seems like a hundred times. Try not to point out that they have already asked the same question. Calmly give them the same answer.

9. Ignore the behavior. If a behavior is not reinforced, it may stop. Do not bring to their attention a behavior that you want to change. If a person is having trouble bathing, instead of saying, "Great job—you didn't refuse your bath today," say, "You had a nice bath today." Keep it positive.

10. Sometimes a person who is anxious might be trying to get your attention. They may feel abandoned or neglected, and so they act out. Try spending some additional time with them.

What you may see or hear or think is not always accurate. As a caregiver, one of the most important things you can do is to look and listen for what is not obvious. A person with dementia who is worried about mealtimes is not concerned about the time—they just want to be fed and cared for. Their repetitive questioning might be because of a communication problem. They are worried and need to be reassured that all is well; they are looking for reassurance. The same thing goes for a person who checks and rechecks their purse, wallet, or the drawers. For a woman, her purse holds her life. A man's wallet means that he is still a provider. An organized dresser drawer means that the person has clean clothes they can wear and that they are able to remain acceptably dressed in society. Constant checking or rummaging is a way to reassure themselves that all is well. Money is a worry for most of us, and so is personal and family safety. The big four in anxiety are the basics: food, shelter, clothing, and family. In order to reduce anxiety and agitation, calmly reassure the person who has dementia through your tone of voice, gentle touch, and actions that they are safe, loved, and respected.

Lesson Eight: *Understanding Wandering*

A person who wanders is trying to locate security. Many people who wander tend to pace. A person will pace out of fear, confusion, or restlessness. Some people who pace are trying to create for themselves some stability or normalcy in their world. Two of my clients come immediately to mind. One was a mail carrier. At the clinic I would do our counseling outside, where he felt most comfortable, and we would talk while walking back and forth in the parking lot. I had another client who would walk the halls of the nursing home. His walking through the halls and into patients' rooms drove the staff crazy until I informed them that he is a retired doctor and that he believed that he was still doing rounds.

A person who has dementia may at some point wander. This means that they no longer recognize the rooms in their home, and they may aimlessly roam through rooms or go outside to find some comfort. There is another side to wandering, a very dangerous side. Wandering means leaving an area by foot, wheelchair, or car and ending up somewhere else. According to recent statistics, in one year over 125,000 people wandered away from their home or from their caregiver. These are just the reported occurrences; the majority of people who wander away never get reported. Approximately 60 percent of people who have dementia will at some time wander away from their home. Of these wanderers, 75 percent will wander repeatedly. If a person who has dementia is not found within twenty-four hours, they might die. Exposure to the elements and dehydration will cause additional confusion. They are no longer able to recognize familiar surroundings such as a street, lake, pond, stream, or ocean, and this unfamiliarity can cause serious injury or death. A person with memory loss will lose their ability to judge the speed of an oncoming car or to recognize a crosswalk. They may walk into traffic. They may not respond to hearing their name.

The perception of a person with dementia is forever changed. They are no longer able to recognize or register what is happening now, which is dangerous. While on a cruise ship one of my clients believed that she was crossing a street to see a friend, and she tried to go over the rail. While the family was watching a show and thought Mom was sound asleep in her cabin, a crew member saw the woman, who had one leg over the railing when he pulled her safely back on deck.

What you or I might consider aimless walking has a purpose for the person who is having memory problems. A person who has dementia may revisit past memories, and these memories blend and meld with their now. In order for you to have a better handle on wandering, there are several things you will need to understand.

1. There are many reasons a person may wander. For some people, wandering may relieve stress or anxiety. For others, wandering may happen because they are searching for something. It can be a familiar person from their past, a place that they once felt safe in, or an object that gave them comfort. Some people, like the mail carrier and the doctor, may be just returning to the safety and structure of their former routines. Some people wander because they are bored.

2. Communication problems may cause wandering. A person may be confused, anxious, hungry, in need of the bathroom, bored, or in pain. Some people

may wander because of their frustration at not being understood.

3. People may wander because they need physical exercise. Many people once had jobs that required them to be active. Being a homemaker meant doing laundry, dusting, sweeping, cooking, and cleaning. A person may wander because of their pent-up energy.

4. Wandering may be caused by environmental factors. A person with dementia may have a problem understanding where they are, have a sense of overload, feel constrained by their clothing or by their environment, be responding to an uncomfortable temperature, or not recognize where they are.

5. A person who feels tension may wander. If they feel that the task is too complicated and they no longer feel capable, they may leave their current surroundings. They may also leave if they feel that they are being treated like a child, are bored with an activity, or are not able to interpret the desires or reactions of the caregiver.

6. Some people just want to go back home. Home is not an actual physical place; it is an emotional place. Home is a where a person feels wanted and loved. Home is a safe place. It's about Mom, Dad, siblings, or even a beloved pet. Home means security. A person with dementia has needs and will search for home— like Dorothy did in *The Wizard of Oz*.

7. Some people wander by accident. They go out to pick up the newspaper or bring in the mail and, once outside, forget their purpose and just keep on going.

One of my clients wandered away from his home after taking out the trash, while another client mistook the front door for the bathroom door.

8. Some people wander away on purpose. I have several clients who told me that for personal reasons they wanted to leave their current home, so they left. Just because they have dementia doesn't mean that they want to stay where they are now. One of my clients, who could not walk and was in a wheelchair, was stopped by the police on the entrance ramp to a major highway. As his family explained to me, "Since Dad was in a wheelchair, we never thought he could leave."

When you are dealing with a person who has dementia, at some point, despite what you may think or believe, they may wander. The following are some things you can do to keep your loved one safe.

- Register with Safe Return through the Alzheimer's Association. They have an identification bracelet or necklace to be worn by the person who has dementia and also one for the caregiver. This jewelry is nationally recognized by law enforcement, paramedics, and many laypersons. The benefit for the caregiver is that if their loved one is lost, wearing this bracelet may save their life and return them where they belong. By wearing the complimentary bracelet as a caregiver, if something happens to you, Safe Return will alert the national hotline that you are caring for a person with memory loss. They will send help to your home or someone on your list to stay with your loved one.

- Always keep on hand a current picture of the person with dementia.

- Remove or change familiar locks to make it difficult or impossible for the person to leave.

- Install a professional security system that chimes, or put bells on the doors that will alert you if a door or window is opened.

- Provide for a safe backyard or front yard space. Buy a pool fence, secure the backyard, and use a lock to control wandering. If the person enjoys sitting on the front porch, place a gate or barrier that will limit their access to the street.

- Check the door knobs. Consider replacing your current door knobs with something that is difficult or different from their current knob. Round door knobs with childproof plastic handles that are easily placed on the existing door knobs work well.

- Disguise the doors. Place a sheet or curtain in front of a door. Out of sight is out of mind.

- Change the level of the lock. If a person is used to using their key at one level changing the location of the lock might stop them from trying to leave. You can also install an additional lock at a different level.

- Use a bean bag chair. These chairs are comfortable to sit in, but for the wanderer they may be difficult to get out of.

- Install safety gates on stairs as a barrier so that the person with dementia will not be able to use the stairs.

- If the person still drives, many states have a "Silver Alert" program, in which the police are contacted if the person is missing. The police send out a missing person report with a picture of the person and the color, make, and model of the car as well as the license plate number.

Wandering often goes unreported. My mother was an unreported wanderer. Actually she was a serial wanderer. She repeatedly left home by foot or car—if she had wings, I'm sure she would have flown off the roof. I never reported her as missing. I now know that I was lucky. I have read reports about incidents in which people turned their back for a second or they took a nap, and their loved one disappeared. I also have many clients who wandered away from religious services, the mall, family gatherings, reunions, holiday parties, and their neighborhood. One of my clients ended up on the local news, having wandered away after services at church. Another person who had dementia was found drowned in her own swimming pool. Through the years of dealing with thousands of people with dementia, the most important lesson I have learned is to never underestimate a person's capabilities. One of my clients was on a locked floor of a day center. Because he looked and appeared normal, nobody noticed when he got on the elevator with another couple who was leaving the floor. He walked past security and was picked up by a good person who offered him a ride. Since he was confused about how to find his way home, they dropped him off at the police station, and the police called his spouse.

People with dementia who wander are disoriented and trying to find their way back home or to a familiar place. They are no longer able to recognize where they are because mentally they are in a different time and place. Where there is a will, there is a way. No matter what you believe or how well you know the person (or even if they are in a wheelchair), at some point in this disorder, a person with dementia has a 60 percent chance of wandering away from home and from you.

Lesson Nine: *Understanding Paranoia*

Put yourself in the shoes of the person who has dementia. Your brain is changing, but you cannot see the changes or recognize that change is happening. As we age, our faces will wrinkle, and our bodies will sag. Our mind sees us one way, and the mirror shows us another. Sad but true: our perception of how we look and the reality of how we look are different. We have been taught at a young age by our parents, family, friends, and the media that strangers can hurt you. To a person who is paranoid and has memory loss, everyone is now a stranger—even themselves. When they see their own face in a mirror or as a shadow in a reflection in a car window, they see a stranger. Over time, a person with dementia will forget familiar people. Family members, friends, and familiar caregivers will eventually become strangers.

Paranoia is fear. A paranoid person has lost their sense of trust and safety. They feel scared, powerless, and insecure. A paranoid person is trying in their own way to make some sense of their current reality. Holding on to their reality allows the person with dementia to have control of their life. It doesn't matter if you as the caregiver or family member feel that the person is being irrational. The person with dementia has one goal: a return to the familiar. Keep this in mind when you are dealing with a paranoid person who truly believes that you have stolen their money, jewelry, or clothing, or are poisoning them, abandoning them, having an affair, or trying to kill them. In their mind, what they think is happening is real to them. Because of the changes in their brain, they will find some way to make sense of their current situation. And once they do, they will hold on to this idea for a very long time. No amount of reality will change what they believe to be true.

Paranoia is a disruptive behavior for caregivers to live with. The best advice I can give you is to find some way not to take any of this behavior personally. Even though you may be the "enemy target" of the person you are caring for, know that the verbal assaults and accusations directed at you are not personal. On the other hand, I have met some caregivers who have used their loved one's memory loss for their own personal or financial gain. In this case the person was not being paranoid: they were right on the money. A person who is paranoid may also have delusions and hallucinations. (A delusion is where a person believes something is true even though it's not. A hallucination is where a person will see, hear, touch, or smell things that aren't there but believe that they are.) So how do you differentiate between a fear of something real and paranoia? Sometimes you can't.

No matter what the truth is or how many reasonable explanations are given, a person who is paranoid will continue to believe what they feel is real. Despite how much you as the caregiver can show them that their belief is false—through concrete evidence, explanations, and clarifications—you will not be heard. No matter what you say or what factual knowledge you present, the paranoid person will continue to believe what they want to believe. A typical example is that if the person hides a piece of jewelry and cannot find it, they now accuse you of stealing the jewelry. Even if you live

1,500 miles away and haven't seen Mom in two years, she will believe and will tell everyone who will listen to her, either in person or by phone, that you stole her jewelry. Her blaming of you may come from something in the past that might have happened with another person or something that you did years ago, and Mom now confuses a past moment with today. Some of my clients tell me that Mom loaned money to a child or grandchild that was never repaid or that jewelry was long ago borrowed and never returned. Mom may have never voiced her displeasure back then and kept her feelings to herself, and now her anger is coming out.

Paranoia has some realistic overtones. When a person has dementia, many of their feelings and memories get jumbled up, and since they no longer live by social constraints, buried feelings come out and become their "now." If years ago you borrowed jewelry, or wanted to borrow jewelry, you may now be accused of stealing it.

A delusion is a paranoid belief that is contrary to a fact. A person who is delusional lives in their own world. Typical delusions are "This is not my home" or "You are not my (spouse or family member)." They may also tell stories that are a mixture of fact and fiction, and what they say sounds plausible. One person may believe that their caregiver is going to abandon them; another may believe that their partner is having an affair. (Some people who no longer recognize their own clothes believe that their spouse is having an affair and that the "other woman" or "other man" is leaving their clothes in the closet or on the bathroom floor.) Delusions will be difficult to deal with when the false accusations are directed at you. The person with dementia appears to outsiders as being normal, rational, and reasonable. Now you are put on the defensive and have to explain to family members and outsiders that none of these accusations are valid.

A paranoid person is no longer capable of separating fact from fiction or accepting reality. There is nothing you can do or say to change a person's mind or response when they are having delusions. The best way to deal with a delusional person is to not take what is happening personally and go about your life as best you can. Some medication and environmental changes may calm a person and their delusions.

A hallucination is a misperception of reality. For the person who has dementia, a hallucination is now their reality. Because of the changes in their brain they may see, hear, feel, or smell something that nobody else does. The person having a hallucination is the only person who is experiencing it. No one else can see what they see, hear what they hear, feel what they feel, or smell what they smell. A hallucination is a personal experience. A person who has dementia will see things; rarely will they hear things. If they do hear something, it typically is a buzzing, tapping, or phone ringing sound. They might hear children or adults who are now "taking over" their home talking. Normally, these voices are people talking among themselves or possibly arguing with the person with dementia. Rarely will a person with dementia hear voices talking to them and telling them to do damage to themselves or others. Voices like that might indicate another disorder such as schizophrenia, a condition that, unless diagnosed in their youth, is rare in the elderly. Many of the hallucinations a person with dementia have are harmless. They may see people in a room or see animals or bugs that are not really there. No matter what they see, or think that they see, it is real to them. As a caregiver, you will need to accept their new reality and find some way to work within this new world.

When your loved one is paranoid, delusional, or hallucinating, you are now going to have to deal with what some consider to be the most difficult and disturbing of all behaviors. The following are some tips, thoughts, and suggestions to help you through this time.

1. The person should have a physical checkup. Infection, dehydration, malnutrition, or medication can cause behavior disorders. Keep in mind that physical illnesses such as infection, pain, fecal impaction, anemia, or respiratory disease can cause changes in behavior.

2. Check for sensory deficits. As we age, our hearing, sight, smell, and taste will change, and so will how we perceive the moment.

3. Review medication. There are many medications whose side effects include hallucinations. A combination of medications may cause delusions and paranoia. Depending on the type of dementia, there are some people who should never take any anti-psychotic medication.

4. A change in the environment may trigger paranoia, delusions, or hallucinations. If a person has recently been moved from their home, gone on a holiday, or has a new caregiver, these changes may be the cause of a behavioral problem.

5. Keep in mind that the removal of items (such as jewelry or money) or taking over the finances may cause a problem. Before you replace the family jewels, have an exact duplication of the jewelry made. I say "exact" because when it comes to jewelry, a person with dementia is hypersensitive and vigilant. They may forget what they did five minutes ago, but they will recognize the difference in weight, color, and clarity of their jewelry pieces.

For many people with paranoia, delusions, and hallucinations, this is just a temporary stage. Eventually it will end. As the brain changes, the behaviors will change. The hallucination or delusion may be disruptive to the family, but in the scheme of life, the behavior is not really harming anyone; in fact, it may be comforting to the person who has dementia.

I had a client, Max, who loved his cat, Morris. He fed him, groomed him, played with him, and watched TV with him on a special chair. Max even slept with Morris. Max is married to Alice. During my consultation with Alice, it turns out that she was so upset with Max's obsession with his imaginary cat that it was driving her over the edge. She was about to leave her husband of fifty-six years over an imaginary cat! Alice wanted me to recommend medication to make the whole Morris the cat thing disappear. After spending some time speaking with Alice, I discovered that what she really wanted was for the whole dementia thing to go away and have back the man she married. After four sessions of educating Alice about dementia and coaching her through her grief of this disorder and her relationship, at their six-month visit Max plopped down in my comfy office chair happy as can be. Alice looked happy too. During the intake I asked several questions (avoiding the questions of hallucinations because of Alice's displeasure over Morris the cat). When Max left the room, I asked Alice about Morris. She told me that the cat was still there (in his mind), but based on my advice, she was living with it. I asked her what changed her attitude. Alice broke out laughing and said that every time she would get upset about the cat, she would remember when I said, "Morris is the perfect pet. He doesn't need to be let out, and there's no litter to be changed, no cat food to buy, and no hair on the furniture."

When it comes to dementia, most hallucinations are harmless. Education and therapy for the caregiver is often much better than giving medicine to stop disruptive behaviors when a person has dementia. There will be times, however, when a person is paranoid, hallucinating, or delusional, and medication and hospitalization are not only necessary but needed. I have known a few individuals who became violent. In all my years in the field, only ten of my clients had to be hospitalized to control their behavior. Some of these institutionalizations could have been avoided, had the families been open to education and counseling. No matter who you are caring for, if you are physically or verbally threatened, or the person you are caring for puts themselves or you at risk of physical harm, they may need to be hospitalized.

Lesson Ten: *Understanding Sundown Syndrome*

For some people who have dementia, as the light changes, their perception and personality change. As the light starts to fade, the person with memory loss may become temporarily anxious, paranoid, or aggressive or start to wander around the home. It's a Dr. Jekyll and Mr. Hyde moment. Keep in mind' that a person who is having memory loss will have additional sensory loss and will become even more confused as daylight starts to decrease. Within minutes or hours, sensory confusion will cause the person to be anxious. Anxiety will kick in, leading to paranoia. When they become fearful, agitation will start. The person who is sundowning will want to go where they feel safe. In their mind, this is the place they call home.

Sundowning is, for lack of a better word, scary for the person who is experiencing it. As the light changes, so does their world. In the changing light, once-familiar objects take on a whole new meaning. Because of their memory and perception problems, the person with dementia will see things differently, because their visual perception has changed. What you might mistakenly believe to be a delusion or hallucination is actually an illusion. For the person with dementia, the light pole outside their house is now a person, or footsteps are an intruder. Shadows become people or animals. For the person who is sundowning, everything they believe is real.

Sundowning is a vicious cycle and once started is hard to stop, but there are ways to deal with it and sometimes avoid it. For caregivers, it is possibly the most disruptive behavior (after paranoia) because it comes on suddenly and then is gone by the next morning, only to start again the next day. It is unrealistic and even futile to try to convince a person who has a memory problem that what they think is real is not. Once a person starts to sundown, the only thing you can do is to provide a safe place for them and tell yourself that tomorrow is another day. I will give you the steps that you can use to avert sundown syndrome, but I have to be honest and tell you that once a person has worked themselves into an agitated sundown mode, there is little that you can do at the time.

For the last several years, I have been studying sundowning. Since sundowning is common in persons who have dementia, I wanted to better understand this disorder. I researched and read published articles about this disorder and how the amount of light affects dementia. It turns out that all of the studies to date show that lack of light or changing light will cause sundowning. One of the reasons I bought my house is that it is so bright. I thought that my mother would be comfortable here, and she was. My house has over thirty-three windows and doors. Forget the cliché: I live in a glass house! So for my personal light experiment I stayed home for one week and sat in the same spot, on the same chair, and watched how the sunlight changed from mid-afternoon to dusk. As the earth rotated, the sunlight changed, and the light in the room shifted. As the day progressed, the room I sat in was still sun bright, but shadows started to form. Familiar items started to look different to me as the light changed. The next week I did the same experiment in my bedroom. The same results held true in my bedroom, which has south, east, and west exposures. The tree in the daylight is just a tree. As the sun light changes, the tree became a Viking warrior who is outside of my bedroom window and is watching me. I may have a vivid imagination, but even without dementia, as the light changed, the tree was scary to me.

Once started, sundowning is difficult to stop, but there are some things that you can do to help decrease its effects.

- In mid-afternoon, turn on all the lights. Yes, you will have an increase in your electric bill, but there will be a decrease in a disruptive behavior. Remember that when we hit age sixty, we need additional light.

- Have the person with dementia sit outside in direct sunlight for at least twenty minutes in the morning. This is not the time to be concerned about skin cancer. They will get a daily dose of Vitamin D when the sun hits their skin. Sunlight helps to reset the circadian rhythm that regulates our sleep-wake cycle and can help reduce behavioral disturbances.

- Try bright light therapy. Many people have Seasonal Affective Disorder (SAD), which is common in the northern states and becoming more recognized even in the southern states, especially during the late fall through springtime.

Because of the shortened day, there is less sunlight. The elderly are especially vulnerable, no matter what the season is, because they rarely spend time outside. Purchase a light box, and have the person use it in the morning for at least forty-five minutes daily. There is some controversy as to which is better—white or blue light. Either may work well, and some studies have shown that after three weeks use, depression was lifted. Anyone with eye disease should consult with an ophthalmologist before using them. Bottom line: get outdoors in sunlight when possible.

- Try to prevent the person with dementia from napping. Waking up from a nap late in the day can cause confusion and lead to sundowning. Some people will confuse 6 AM with 6 PM.

- Check medication. A medication that is given earlier in the day may cause later disorientation.

- Rule out discomfort. A person who has dementia may not be able to tell you what is causing them pain. Clothing that fit well in the morning may be uncomfortable later in the day.

- Avoid anything that has caffeine after the morning hours. Caffeine may cause anxiety, which for some people may add to sundowning.

- Encourage daytime activity. The more active a person is in daytime, the more tired they will be, and they may not notice the light change.

- Keep the person engaged. Have the person be an active participant in preparing a meal or setting the table.

- Shut off the TV.

- Use diversion. Give the person with dementia an activity that they are capable of doing, and then let them do it.

- Focus and refocus a person with dementia to stay on their task.

- Go for an outing. If possible, go out for ice cream, a car ride, or a short visit to a friend's or neighbor's home that involves a sweet treat. Sometimes a nice diversion can stop sundowning. When you come home, immediately start their bedtime routine.

- If a person is sundowning, don't wait to give them medication after they have worked themselves into an agitated moment. If Mom is in a current pattern of sundowning at 4 PM, ask her doctor if you can give her medication at an earlier time. The medication will take time to work. Always consult with the doctor before changing a dose or time.

- Keep to a schedule. A person who has any form of dementia should have a routine. A person with dementia needs structure to feel safe, and structure helps avoid sundowning. Routines are safe, predictable, and naturally calming. For my clients who have a routine, sundowning rarely happens, and they have reduced difficult behaviors.

- Remain calm. If you get upset, the person with dementia will mirror your reaction, which will increase their agitation. Try not to reason; instead reassure. Validate the person's concerns. Use positive words.

- Provide reassurance. Walk and talk through what is happening. Validate the person who has memory loss. If they are trying to go back home, instead of saying, "This is your home," ask them about their home. When a person says that they have to go home to take care of the children, instead of saying that their children are grown, ask them about their children. To be successful when you are dealing with a person who is sundowning, you will have to be in the moment—their moment.

- Keep in mind that, despite your best efforts, medication might be needed to get through this period. The use of medication should be monitored and used only on a short-term basis.

- Ask your doctor about adding Vitamin D in pill form if the person is sunlight-deficient.

Nobody knows why sundowning happens. I have asked many of my clients in their better moments to tell me why sundowning occurs and what happens to them during those moments. Their answer is they don't know or they can't control themselves. To reduce the behavior of sundowning, I have found that keeping a log may be helpful. Record what the person does during the day, what they ate, what was on TV, and other details of their day. The purpose of the log is to track certain times or events that may trigger the sundowning episodes. Remember, a person who has dementia is now in a different place and time in their mind. The five o'clock news can be the trigger; a clock can be too. Evenings can be the trigger to times in their past that their children, spouse, or they themselves needed to be home. Review the log, and note the time the behavior starts and what occurs. This will help you to recognize what causes a behavior and how to stop it before it happens.

Lesson Eleven: *Understanding Aggressiveness*

Let's face it: we all have days where nothing seems to go right. The car doesn't start, we are late to work, the boss has an attitude, clients are unreasonable, on the way home traffic is ridiculous, and when you finally get home, you are bombarded by problems and bills. After a big rain the new roof leaks; your son is flunking math, and your daughter needs braces; the dog needs to be walked, the garbage hasn't been taken out, and dinner still needs to be made. The dinner hour is now a war zone. Everyone is eating and complaining, sniping at each other, and after someone says, "I'm not going to eat this," you explode. Once you explode, everyone thinks that you have lost your mind. I call this the "volcanic effect." There is only so much that any one person can take before they lose it, and it may seem that the person loses control over the smallest thing. The reality is that life is stressful and filled with constant demands. Like a volcano that slowly builds, most of us can handle the daily stuff that is thrown at us until we hit the point where we erupt. For some of us, there comes a point in time when if Mother Teresa lived our stressful life, even she would lose her composure.

A volcanic response is normal. Our lives are stressful and filled with so many responsibilities and concerns that it is totally normal to occasionally explode and get all of our emotions out. An explosion is a good thing. If you hold all of your emotions in, you might risk a major heart attack or a stroke. After a volcanic episode, a normally rational person will calm down and recognize that it's just a bad day (or a series of bad days), and they are able to explain to their family the reason for their outburst and apologize for their behavior. Your reaction can now be put in perspective. It can be understood because you have the ability to explain why the outburst happened. Even rational people will have volcanic moments.

For the person who has some form of memory loss, any moment can start a chain reaction that can lead to a bad day and a volcanic moment. The day may start off great and everything is going well, until you remind your loved one that it's time to wake from their nap, get out of bed, bathe, eat, sleep, or go to a doctor's appointment. Suddenly it seems that—out of nowhere—the chaos begins. The person becomes argumentative, stubborn, belligerent, or combative. This is when caregivers frantically put in a call to the doctor's office requesting medication to control this new unwanted behavior. A majority of doctors will immediately prescribe medication to get the situation under control and to stop the caregiver from calling again.

Medication can be helpful in some situations, but the majority of disruptive behaviors are a direct result of actions by the caregiver. Many of the medications typically used for behavioral purposes are not helpful and often cause additional problems. A well-trained and educated caregiver can be the best medicine.

Aggressiveness is often the result of communication gone wrong. Since the brain pathways are no longer working the way they once were, for a person with dementia, life is now frightening, confusing, and frustrating. A person with dementia is no longer able to deal with or understand the current environment. They feel threatened. In order to help keep a person with dementia in a safe physical and emotional place, it will be up to you to make adjustments in their life.

There are various possible causes of aggressiveness in people with dementia:

- overstimulation or the pressure to do things beyond their capabilities

- exhaustion or fatigue

- a new routine—this can mean any change to familiar surroundings

- a change in appetite can trigger aggressive behavior—for some people, their blood sugar may be low, and the lack of food combined even with the usual dosage of medication can cause a behavioral problem

- lack of sleep

- sundowning

- watching the news or a violent TV show

- alcohol

- a personality disorder, either in the person with dementia or in the caregiver

Here is a list and some suggestions that as a caregiver you should keep in mind when coping with aggression:

- Not everyone is naturally nice. Niceness for some people is a learned behavior in order to fit in to society. Many people use the social mask to be accepted. When dementia strikes, the personality you see and experience will often be their true self.

- Do not take any of their behaviors, accusations, or actions personally. A person with dementia will not act appropriately; often times they are in survival mode and want to return to the familiar. A person with dementia will relive past experiences and relieve their stress by letting it out on you. They are now living in the moment, and you just happen to be there.

- Get a medical checkup. Sudden aggressiveness can be a sign of a physical disorder. They may have a urinary tract infection or be constipated. The person may have fallen and have a bruised muscle or a broken bone. If a person has any sudden change in behavior or personality, check with their primary doctor.

- Investigate the medications they are taking. A side effect of some medication is aggressiveness. If they have recently added a new prescription, this could be the cause of the problem. Keep in mind that our body chemistry changes every twenty-four hours; what was tolerated yesterday may not be tolerated today. Every medication will have a different effect on each person who takes it.

- Your approach can either trigger or diffuse aggression. As a caregiver, your behavior in this situation is important. Your frustration and anger can add fuel to the fire. A person who has memory loss will sense your emotions and adopt them as their own.

The following are a few suggestions to protect you if a person becomes aggressive:

- Keep out of harm's way. If the person becomes physically aggressive, your best defense is to stand back. Do not approach them.

- If possible, leave the room. Do not try to reason with the person or argue; this will only confuse them and often make them more determined to defend themselves.

- Get to a phone, and call for support. There may be a family member, neighbor, or clergy who has a special relationship with the person who has dementia, and one of them may be able to calm the person down and ease the situation.

- If the situation doesn't resolve, or if at any time you feel that either you or the person who has dementia is in danger, call 911. An unfamiliar uniformed person such as the police, a security guard, or an EMT (an emergency medical technician or ambulance staff) may calm down the situation. Hopefully, they have been trained to deal with this situation.

- If a person puts your safety or theirs at risk, the Baker Act may apply. The person will be placed in an institution against their will for three days and observed by professionals to determine if they are at a risk to harm themselves or others. They will be in a psychiatric unit, and their medications will be adjusted. If a person is out of control, at this time, as difficult or uncomfortable that this may be for you, this is the best place for them.

- Remove or lock up all weapons, including guns, bows, and knives. If a firearm needs to remain in the home for security reasons, separate the ammunition from the weapon.

Lesson Twelve: *Understanding Sleep Disorders*

Sleep is a time of rejuvenation. While we sleep, we recharge our internal batteries that give us the strength and fortitude to make it through the next day. Sleep is no different from food or medication, yet it is often taken for granted—until we lack it. Without a good night's sleep, we will not function properly. The necessary sleep time for each person will vary. Some people need more sleep; others can function well on less. As we age our sleep time will change as well as our quality of sleep. As we age, the quality of our sleep changes. Some of us wake up frequently for bathroom breaks, or due to pain, or anxiety and this will disrupt our sleep. For most people, to function at their best, they will need to have anywhere from six to nine hours nightly of quality sleep time. I know for me to operate at 100 percent, I need eight hours of sleep. After a hard day, I may need nine hours of sleep to recharge. With anything less, the next day, I'm not operating on all cylinders. Without a good night's sleep, I don't perform well the next day. When a person is sleep deprived for just one night, their functioning will be as if they drank two cocktails. When you lose sleep for two days, you might as well have four cocktails.

Most caregivers and people with dementia will suffer from some form of sleep disorder at some time. As we age, our sleep times will change, and the quantity of our sleep changes during our lifespan. Babies spend two-thirds of their days sleeping (and so do teenagers), while adults spend just one-third of their day sleeping. The quality of our sleep will change too. Stress, anxiety, and depression will affect sleep. So will additional aging problems such as changes in our hormones, urinary frequency, arthritis, restless leg syndrome, toothache, constipation, or an ingrown toenail, all of which may cause difficulty in either falling or staying asleep. A confusing or new environment may cause sleep problems. Listening to a person snore will cause a caregiver a sleep problem. Clothing may cause a sleep problem.

The amount of sleep we need will vary depending on our age, environment, responsibilities, and circadian rhythm. As a parent and a caregiver, I know firsthand about sleep deprivation. Caring for a newborn is a walk in the park compared to caring for a person with dementia, especially a person who now has problems sleeping. If the person you're caring for has problems sleeping, so will you. Lack of sleep will eventually affect your job and your relationships. Caring for a person who spends their nights wandering through the home is disruptive. Lack of sleep will make it harder to focus on the rest of your responsibilities. You may stop attending social functions because you are too tired, or you may have problems functioning at your job, maintaining your relationships, or caring for your family. A person who is sleep-deprived will have difficulty functioning, and this will add to behavior problems.

I know what it is like to have my sleep interrupted because of caring for another person. Remember earlier when I said that I need eight hours of sleep? Actually, I need more to make up for all the years I cared for my children and parents. The loss of sleep I had from my two children was expected; spending my nights awake following my mother around the house and keeping her safe wasn't expected and was more upsetting because nobody understood what I was going through. It's expected that children will grow out of their sleep problems—it's temporary and normal. As for adults with dementia, sleep problems can continue for years.

Two of the biggest complaints I hear from caregivers is that a person is either sleeping too little (insomnia) or sleeping too much (hypersomnia). The more you know about sleep and sleep disorders, the better you will be able to deal with the person who has dementia. Here are some steps to take if your loved one is having sleep problems:

1. Rule out any medical problems. If a person is uncomfortable, sleep will be interrupted or impossible.

2. Review medication. Some medications can cause a person to lose sleep or sleep too much.

3. Remove stimulants such as caffeine and sugar as well as heavy meals before bedtime.

4. Have the person reduce their intake of liquids in the evening.

5. Eliminate, reduce, or water down alcoholic beverages they consume. Alcohol will affect sleep.

6. Check the bedroom temperature. Each of us has a personal comfort zone. Adjust the temperature on the thermostat, or change the bedding to provide for warmth or coolness.

7. Ensure that the person uses good sleep hygiene. Be consistent, and keep to a routine. This means a regular bedtime, possibly a foot or body massage, and reading

a book or watching a nonviolent or not stimulating TV show. Avoid the news channels.

8. Reduce stimulation. Make the bedroom area a sanctuary. Reduce lighting. Deflect outside noise by playing comforting, soothing music. Heavy curtains can reduce outside light and provide a noise barrier.

9. Give reassurance. In a calm tone, tell the person with dementia that it is time to go to sleep and that you will be lying either next to them or in a nearby room. Tell them that it is safe to go asleep. If they feel the need to check the doors, accompany them, and talk them through this step. Instead of saying, "Mom, we have checked the doors twelve times—let's go to sleep," say, "Mom, I feel so much safer that you want to make sure that all of the doors are locked. After we check the doors together, we will be able to go to sleep."

10. Depending on what their normal routine was before the person had dementia, they may enjoy or look forward to a walk around the block or a short drive in the car to help them sleep better.

11. If possible, try to discourage daytime napping. Encourage daytime activities.

12. Sunlight will help reset a person's natural sleep-wake cycle. Have the person with dementia spend at least fifteen minutes in the morning sunlight. Try bright light therapy in the morning hours, especially if you live in the north or during the rainy season in the south.

13. Keep anything stressful to a minimum.

14. If a person is sleeping too much, try to establish a routine in which they will have scheduled activities such as physical therapy, day center, exercise, or another purpose to get them out of bed.

15. Check the mattress. Many people have bedding that is uncomfortable. A mattress is not a family heirloom. The mattress should be replaced every seven to ten years. Consider buying an encased mattress cover to reduce dust mites and bed bugs. This covering will also protect the mattress from moisture.

16. The same thing applies to pillows. Over time, pillows can become uncomfortable and will need to be replaced. Buy new ones, and purchase pillow coverings.

17. Check clothing. Some bed time clothing may be too constraining or uncomfortable. For some people, the less clothes the better; others may prefer more coverage. Consider taking off the person's jewelry and placing the items on the nightstand table. Jewelry worn at night may cause a sleep disturbance.

18. Hospital beds are not a physical restraint or a deterrent. Many accidents occur when a person who has dementia tries to get over the rails or scoots out of a hospital bed.

19. Consider hiring a night aide for a short time so that you can catch up on your sleep.

A Cheat Sheet on Disruptive Behaviors

Always keep in mind that the person with dementia is having involuntary changes to their brain that are causing them to act or react in certain ways. They are powerless to control themselves and their emotions. This is not who they once were, or who they would like to be, but because of the changes in their brain, this is who they are now. Remember: no matter what the behavior, there is still a viable person inside. The reason for their reaction is that they are not being heard or understood, or their needs are being ignored. They are now frustrated and want to get their needs met, and as a caregiver you want your own needs met.

Some disruptive behaviors happen because a person who was once self-sufficient is now having difficulty caring for themselves. They may lose the ability to speak for themselves. When additional help is forced on them, they may react with anger, rage, frustration, and depression. This is where you come in. You never wanted this job, but, then again, most adults would not have dreamed that they would have to depend on the care of others to live—especially the care from a spouse or a child.

In order to avoid a disruptive behavior and to deal successfully with a person who has dementia, you will need to keep the following in mind:

1. Changes to the brain will cause a person to act differently.

2. As the disease progresses, a person will lose their ability not only to verbally communicate with you but to understand what you are saying and be able to do the tasks that you ask them to do.

3. Home is safe. Anything outside of home is now a personal threat or frightening. A person who has dementia does not want to leave the safety of their home.

4. Incontinence is a real concern. Being able to go to the bathroom or the thought that they might not find a bathroom will keep many people homebound. It may also cause anxiety, agitation, and isolation.

5. Education about this disorder, not medication, is often the best prescription. Medication is good and sometimes great, but for some people and some types of dementia medication may cause additional physical and behavioral problems.

6. Accept and deal with the reality of the now, instead of clinging to your dreams of how the future should be.

7. Know that any behavior is just a phase. Behaviors do not last forever.

8. Reevaluate medication, especially medication that is prescribed for a challenging behavior, every three months.

9. Have the person evaluated for food allergies.

10. Check for any discomfort such as pain or illness. When in doubt, call 911.

11. Realize that some behaviors may be caused by hunger, thirst, pain, or fatigue.

12. Everybody responds to touch. When was the last time you touched your loved one?

13. Prescribed medication can have a different effect than what was intended. Some medications can cause hallucinations, memory loss, depression, anxiety, or fatigue.

14. Try to create a safe, calming environment. Look for things that may be frightening or distressing to the person with dementia. Put yourself in their shoes and readjust the environment.

15. Be aware of your tone of voice. Your tone will make a difference, creating a calm situation or a volcanic reaction.

16. Provide a dependable routine that includes meals, snacks, fluids, and a bedtime schedule.

17. Keep the person with dementia clean, dry, and comfortable.

18. Play relaxing and appropriate music for the person with dementia.

19. Watch your emotions. Be soft. Speak softly; move softly. Try not to have sudden movements or short words. If you are angry, frustrated, or tired, they may mirror your emotions. Try to be positive and upbeat. A person with dementia may not understand what you are saying, but they can read your emotions.

20. Have something on hand for a distraction. Give the person something tangible to hold onto, play with, or chew on. If possible, try to distract them with a reward such as an outing, a snack, or an activity that they enjoy.

21. Try not to point out the behavior you want to stop. Instead, encourage good behavior by validating successful moments. Encourage instead of discourage. Point out the positives. Instead of saying, "You forgot to put forks on the dinner table," say, "Mom, you set

the table beautifully." Instead of saying, "Mom, the doctor said that you need to exercise more," when she has walked seven steps, say, "Mom, I'm proud of you. You did a great job walking today."

Above all, keep in mind that you are dealing with a human being. Just because they are having difficulty communicating or understanding what is expected of them does not make them less human. A person having a problem with their memory doesn't mean that you can take advantage of them or ignore their feelings. A person with dementia might not be able to communicate their needs, but they will have moments of clarity. No matter what stage of dementia they are in, they are still capable of making their needs known. We may call their actions "disruptive behaviors" or "challenging behaviors," but they are just trying to get their needs met. As a caregiver, your job is to watch, listen, and take action. The bottom line is that most disruptive behaviors are a result of unmet needs; since the person is no longer able to say what they want, they will physically or emotionally act out. It will be up to you, the caregiver, to figure out how to make both of your lives better.

CHAPTER NINE

HOME SAFETY

As we age, our senses will change over the course of time. Our vision, as well as sense of smell, taste, and touch, will diminish. As we get older, some of us may look great on the outside, but there are certain physiological conditions we cannot escape. According to research, the majority of sixty-year-olds will experience:

- Loss of vision. A person over sixty will need three times the amount of light to see as well as they did when they were younger.

- Loss of taste buds. Most people over sixty will have lost 50 percent of their taste buds. A person in their seventies has one-sixth of the taste buds of a twenty-year-old.

- Loss of sense of smell. After age sixty, a person's sense of smell may dramatically diminish.

- Loss of sense of touch. The brain sends out fewer signals to the fingers as a person ages, so they will not be able to feel objects or even themselves the same way they did when they were younger.

- Loss of hearing. Many people suffer needlessly from an undiagnosed hearing loss. Keep in mind that you cannot remember what you do not hear.

When you put into perspective the normal losses that occur during aging, and then take into account memory loss for a person with dementia, a once safe environment can become a safety concern. Keep in mind that over time a person with dementia will lose their ability to:

- recognize everyday familiar objects
- get started on a task
- stay focused on a task
- put steps in a logical order
- follow directions

Safety in the home environment is often the most overlooked issue for people with memory loss. Ensuring a safe home can increase the quality of life and reduce disruptive behaviors for people with dementia. Most doctors do not give a prescription for home environment safety. Doctors are often not aware of the importance that the role the environment plays or of how home life affects the person with dementia and their caregivers. Some doctors may write a prescription for medication and then send the patient home. What many doctors and families fail to realize is that home may not be the best place for the person with memory loss unless the house is made safe. The goal of home safety is to reduce accidents, provide a stress-free environment for both the person with dementia and their caregivers, encourage mobility and stimulation, create a sense of personal safety, increase quality of life, and reduce inappropriate or disruptive behaviors.

It may sound simple, but a safe home is a happy home. A safe home may mean the person will need less or no medication. The following are ten key points to keep in mind when ensuring a safe environment for a person with dementia:

1. People over the age of fifty will start to experience an increased sensitivity to light and glare. Glare is often blinding and is the main reason that many people no longer enjoy being outdoors. Indoors, it is best to use window treatments such as drapes, shades, or blinds that can be opened to allow light in. Avoid using dark window film treatments, which can give the impression that the outside weather is dark and gloomy. At night, film treatments act like mirrors that can cause agitation and confusion to the person with dementia because they may see their reflection and not recognize themselves. For the outside of the home or patio, try to avoid white walkways. Instead, paint the walkway or patio in a muted shade, or install pavers with grass for contrast to reduce the glare.

2. The outside areas should be inviting. To encourage stimulation and interaction, plant colorful plants, put out bird feeders, use weather vanes, and hang wind chimes. If possible, install a small fountain, and add some Koi or goldfish to provide stimulation, conversation, and activity such as caring for and counting the fish. If you have space in the backyard, place a bench under a shaded tree or an umbrella to encourage being outdoors. Provide a smooth walkway surface that has a loop or a bench to help people turn around and enjoy being outdoors. Depending on where you live or the season, apply bug spray to their clothing or purchase an outdoor fan to discourage mosquitoes and other flying pests.

3. Reduce clothing choices. A full closet is a confusing closet. Pack, throw out, or give away clothing that is no longer worn. Many of us are "pack rats" and keep

clothing that no longer fit properly, has stains, or is no longer appropriate or necessary—think fur coats in Miami. As we age, our bodies change. Clothes may fit differently. For some people, clothing may become too loose, and for others the clothing may be too tight. Ill-fitting clothing can cause accidents and unwanted behaviors.

4. Turn down the volume. Each of us has a personal sensitivity to sound. What sounds good to you may cause another person discomfort. For a person with dementia, sound may trigger disruptive behaviors. If you need to have the TV, radio, or stereo volume turned up high, use headphones.

5. Scent is personal. Each of us has a favorite scent. Our sense of smell is the most primal of all of our senses. Smell is a knee-jerk reaction: it can trigger happiness or despair. Smell triggers emotions. Emotions trigger behaviors. Having grown up by the ocean, I love the smell of the sea water. But I am probably the only person on the planet who for no reason hates the smell of a very popular soap. Some scents can be calming, and others can trigger disrupted behavior. For example, if Mom was abusive and cleaned the home with a strong pine-scented cleanser, this odor may cause an unwanted behavior- Mom may be calmed, but as a caregiver the pine smell will be upsetting to you. In some situations the opposite may occur- Mom gets upset from the Pine smell and as a caregiver you feel calmer.

6. Touch and personal space define an individual's comfort zone. According to the experts, a comfortable

space between people—especially strangers—is an arm's length away (at least in American culture). Some people like closeness; others don't. Always respect and take into consideration the amount of personal space that a person needs to feel comfortable.

7. Taste is personal. The old adage goes: "If it tastes good, eat it." As we age, our taste buds become less sensitive. Food no longer tastes the same. You may need to add more salt or sugar to the meals of a person with dementia to help meet their changing taste buds. On the other hand, some of us will automatically add salt or sugar to our food before ever tasting it. If the person with dementia instantly goes for the salt shaker, avoid adding salt while cooking.

8. Food can be medication. Each of us has a comfort food that brings us back to a memory of home and safety. I have one friend who craves chocolate, another who loves ice cream, one who will kill for Italian food, and me, I love a good salad—I always have, ever since I was eleven years old. During different stages of our lives, our food preferences will change. If you're unsure of what the person likes, go back to the basics —perhaps meatloaf, macaroni and cheese, peanut butter and jelly, oatmeal, and eggs—and experiment from there. Keep in mind that people from different cultures will like different foods.

9. Keep it light. A light-deprived person is a depressed person. Turn on the lights, and during the daytime get them outdoors. People who are exposed to natural sunlight feel better, act better, and sleep better. As a caregiver, do whatever you have to do to get the

person outside for at least forty minutes a day. Walk with them; if they use a wheelchair, wheel them around. Just get them outside. Numerous studies have shown that a person exposed to direct sunlight in the morning will feel and sleep better. When a person is deprived of natural sunlight, their internal body clock malfunctions. Sunlight provides vitamin D, a building block for stronger bones and better sleep.

10. Maintain dignity. Always keep in mind that you are dealing with a person who has their own particular wants and needs. Above all, always respect them and their wishes. Just because they have lost their memory does not mean that they have lost their mind. Remember that the person who you are dealing with is still a person. Overtime, dementia may rob a person of their memories, but dementia will never take away their self.

A person with dementia thinks and lives in the "now" moment. If a light bulb goes out, they will use a step stool or chair or get on the table to change it. There may be an item that they need on a high shelf in the kitchen or closet. How are they going to reach it? By using a ladder, step stool, cabinet, or chair. When a person has dementia, common sense and statistics mean nothing, but they will to you. According to the National Safety Council:

- Each year, 1.8 million Americans over age sixty-five are injured in falls.

- Each year over 8 million home injuries result in a disability. This means that 8 million people need the care of a family member or will need to be placed in a physical rehabilitation unit or nursing home to help them get through their day. And every year 33,000 people die from accidental injuries in their home.

- Every sixteen minutes someone will have an accident at home that will cause their death.

- Every four seconds a disabling injury occurs.

- Each year falls result in the deaths of 8,000 people. It doesn't matter whether they fell off a roof, a ladder, or a step stool or tripped over a rug—a fall is a fall.

The purpose of environmental safety is to:

- Allow a person to stay in their home longer.

- Reduce the risk of accidents that could be fatal or could cause a disability.

- Increase the person's physical and emotional safety, which allows for their increased independence.

- Help the person with dementia maintain their sense of self and control over their environment, which will reduce disruptive behaviors.

- Reduce caregiver stress. Any unwanted behavior that you can stop or prevent will significantly reduce your stress.

The goal of environmental adaptation is to increase the independence of the person with dementia and to reduce the amount of care you need to provide. As the disease progresses, a person with dementia will begin to have difficulty in their environment. The "person in the environment" approach takes into consideration both the person with dementia and the caregiver's needs. It emphasizes the person's social and physical capabilities as well as how they were functioning before their memory loss and how they are functioning now. Environmental changes can help slow the rate of memory loss.

As people age, they become more dependent on their environment to compensate for their increased physical and sensory loss. Home means a safe place, which is why many people want to stay in their home. To the person who is having trouble with their memory, home is the safest place to be. As time goes on and their memory fades, dementia can make any home into an unsafe home.

Keep in mind that different stages of this disease will require you to use different interventions. There is no "one size fits all." Dementia stages are just a guide; each person is going to act differently because of their education, personality, lifestyle, and medical problems. How you personally deal with the person and the situation will matter.

You can make changes to the current environment that will make a world of difference in your life and in the quality of life of the person with dementia. With these changes life will be more manageable.

Lesson One: *Home Safety for the Person with MCI or Mild Dementia*

When a person is diagnosed with MCI (mild cognitive impairment) or with mild dementia, you need to keep in mind that this person is still high-functioning. For the most part, other than some short-term memory loss, almost all of the recently diagnosed will continue to do what they already do. And most live their lives without any difficulties. They will and can continue to work, handle their finances, and be able to drive without any major problems. However, some people who fall into this category need some help. Keep in mind that everyone is unique; the fact that others with the same diagnosis are capable does not always mean that your loved one is too. The environmental changes you can make will benefit the current and future quality of life for both you and the person you are caring for.

1. Install automatic faucet controls. The sensor ensure that the water will only turn on if someone's hands are in front of the faucet and will automatically shut off once they remove their hands. You will no longer have to worry about turning off the water. There are automatic faucets for both kitchen and bathroom sinks.

2. Have a professional alarm system installed that will alert you when a door or window is opened or closed.

3. Place grab bars in the bathroom—especially in the shower. If possible, place one across from or next to the toilet.

4. Instead of using a step stool, buy a reacher. A reacher is a mechanical claw that can grab things off a shelf. Don't let the simplicity of this device fool you. It allows the person to take off, or put on, items on a shelf without having to climb up on a chair or step stool.

5. Keep spare keys handy. Misplacing keys causes stress. Lost keys are eventually found. To reduce stress, have several spare keys readily available. Keep all the key chain colors the same. People with memory loss do not

want just a set of keys; they want *their* keys. Keeping all the sets identical will avoid many arguments and confusion. You can also buy a battery-operated key locator from an electronics store that with a push of a button will send an electronic sound that will locate the missing keys.

6. If you have a solid door, install a peep hole. Always look through it before you answer the door. Never assume that because you live in a guarded building, the person who is ringing you doorbell is a friend or a neighbor.

7. Install hooks or pegboards for keys at the front door. This also works well for purses. Now is the perfect time to start putting keys or any valuables in one place so that they can easily be located.

8. Install nonslip strips in the bathroom, especially in the tub or shower, and even on the floor around the shower. If the home has stairs, buy reflective strips, and place them on the steps.

9. Lower the water temperature. If the person lives in their own home, set the water heater to read below 110 degrees. If the person lives in an apartment, buy an anti-scald device.

10. Purchase a picture phone. This will allow for one-touch dialing, and the pictures will help the caller recognize whom they want to call.

11. Use a week-long pill box. It only needs to be filled once a week, and all of the medications will be accounted for.

12. Fill the home with bright light. Light reduces depression and other unwanted behaviors. It also makes it easier to see where you are going, and that can reduce falls and confusion.

13. Keep a fire extinguisher handy, and know how to use it. A kitchen fire can start suddenly. Always be prepared.

14. If the person is still using the stove, purchase a device that will automatically shut off the stove at a preset time when the sensor determines that no one is near the stove.

15. Start reducing the clutter. Remove things from the home that may cause confusion. Try to get to the mail early and discard everything that is not important. Throw out all reading material that is not being used. Go through the bathroom, and remove all of the unused or unnecessary products, including medication. Think of it as spring cleaning.

16. Discuss using a Safe Return bracelet. A Safe Return bracelet or necklace will help to identify a person who has dementia. It is universally recognized by police, hospitals, paramedics, and the informed public as a symbol that the wearer has a form of dementia, and it will help reunite a person who is lost with their caregiver. Safe Return also has a companion bracelet that the caregiver can and should wear. If the caregiver is in an accident or is brought to the emergency room, this identification will alert the authorities that the person is caring for someone with dementia. They will then inform Safe Return, who will call backup caregivers from the emergency contact list. Keep in mind that 60 percent of people with dementia will,

at some point, wander off. Many who wander off or get lost for short periods are not reported. I also have clients who tell me that when they got lost, their family had no knowledge of it. The Safe Return bracelet will also be helpful to avoid being arrested. Some people with dementia can have behavioral problems such as aggression, or when confused or agitated they may appear to be under the influence of alcohol or drugs. Some people with dementia will leave a store with items and forget to pay. The Safe Return bracelet informs other people that the wearer has a memory problem. Using it may avoid a trip to the local police station.

17. Now is the time to buy a personal emergency response system (PER). If a person falls, is injured, or needs help, all they have to do is press a button, and they will be instantly connected to a twenty-four-hour emergency response system. This will give peace of mind to both you and the person with dementia.

18. If the person lives in a house, install outdoor lighting. Make sure that all of the walkways are cleared of any debris such as leaves, snow, or water, which can cause falls. If there are outside steps, install reflective nonskid strips. Also, place handrails on both sides of the steps to avoid accidents.

19. Use technology to your advantage. Consider replacing your cell phones with the newer versions that come with a global positioning system (GPS) so that you will be able to locate your loved one. If the person is driving, there are devices that you can purchase and

place in the car that will track their position and how they are driving.

Lesson Two: *Home Safety for the Person with Moderate Dementia*

As the dementia progresses into the moderate stage, there are certain environmental changes you can make that will benefit both you and the person with dementia. Different rooms in the home will call for different changes; the living room, kitchen, bathroom, and bedroom will need to be modified to help the person with dementia remain independent and safe.

The following are tips for making the living room safe for a person in the moderate stage of dementia:

1. Remove clutter. Clear out anything that is no longer necessary or doesn't serve a purpose. Remove all glass objects from tables. Put all incoming mail in a box or bag to remove it from sight. Consider getting a post office box and picking up the mail at the post office. Out of sight is out of mind. Many people who have memory problems become hoarders. Slowly and carefully remove papers from their home. Keep in mind that the person who has dementia may have important documents that are now heaped in the pile of magazines and sweepstakes entries. Carefully go through their papers before you discard them.

2. Check rugs and flooring. Many common area rugs can cause a person with dementia to trip and fall because the person is no longer able to gauge the slight difference in carpet height. Shiny waxed floors are perceived now as wet floors. A person with dementia will often avoid walking on a shiny floor. Another problem is the popular checkerboard floor. For a

person with dementia, the dark or black part of the floor may appear as a dark hole. People with dementia will seldom walk over anything that is dark. The color change will stop them from walking because they think that they will fall into a hole.

3. Keep pathways clear. Home interior design encourages furniture placement that is esthetically pleasing but doesn't always work well for a person with memory loss. A professionally decorated room may look great and work well for you, but for the person with moderate dementia this room can be an obstacle or become a confusing area that will cause additional stress. It is important to have clear pathways so that the person will be able to walk by themselves or with assistance to their destination without having to navigate around furniture. Place the chair or the sofa so that the person can easily see it, walk to it, and then sit down. For the person who has memory loss, they may have a moment when they forget what a sofa is, and walking into the back of a piece of furniture will only add to their confusion and frustration. Arrange the furniture so that it is recognizable and inviting to them.

4. Keep areas well lit and bright. Shadows can cause confusion because of the changed perception and reduced vision of a person who has memory problems. Keep in mind that a person with dementia may no longer be able to separate imagination from reality. As the light changes, so will their feelings of safety and security. What might be light and comfortable for the caregiver may be different for the person with dementia. Reduced light may mean an increase in difficult behaviors. Increase indoor lighting at midday.

5. Put away anything decorative that resembles food. Many of us have glass, plastic, or wooden items that look like fruit or candy. A person with memory loss will no longer be able to understand that these are just objects, and they may try to eat them. To avoid confusion and future dental bills (or possible choking), remove these items.

6. If you have stairs or steps between floors, install hand rails on both sides of the stairs where possible. You want to make sure that the person with dementia has something to hold onto with either hand. If you do not want them to go up or down a flight of stairs, install a gate. Keep in mind that a person with dementia may climb over a gate if they want to go up or down. This can cause a fall. I usually suggest to families that, as a temporary measure, they have a professional install a four- or five-foot-high gate either at the top or at the bottom of the stairway or in both places. This is only a temporary measure. It may not look great, but your goal at this point is for the safety of the person with dementia. Once the person stops wanting to or is no longer able to use the stairs, the gate can be removed.

7. If the bedrooms are on the second floor, consider installing an electric seat chair to move them safely between floors.

To make the kitchen safer for a person with moderate dementia, here are some suggestions:

1. Remove all small appliances that are no longer used on a daily basis. A person with dementia may become confused, agitated, aggressive, or frustrated with

appliances that they can no longer recognize. Put the blender, deep fryer, bread maker, waffle machine, and so forth in a cabinet or in the garage. Out of sight means out of mind. Out of mind means a reduction in unwanted behaviors.

2. Install childproof locks on cabinets, drawers, and, in the case of uncontrollable eating, on the refrigerator. There are also locks that you can place on the oven door. The main goal is to keep a person safe in this stage of memory loss. When they are safe, you get the bonus of maintaining your own sanity. This may mean locking up the glassware, food, cleaning supplies, and knives. Many hardware shops and toy stores carry childproof locks. They are simple to install yourself, or you can hire someone to install them for you. You are now child-proofing in reverse—actually, you are dementia-proofing. The person with moderate dementia, because of changes to their brain, will no longer be able to open cabinets or drawers that have childproof locks on them. Once the kitchen is secured, you will have less to worry about when the person with dementia wanders into the kitchen.

3. Do not wax the floors. For the person with dementia, a shiny floor looks like a wet floor, and they will avoid walking on it. Wet floors mean falls. Falls are terrifying. Many people believe that if they fall, they will break a bone and need surgery, and then spend the rest of their life in a nursing home. People in nursing homes die. Translation: Falls mean death. A person with dementia would rather risk starvation than walk on a shiny floor. Sneakers may stop a person from slipping, but they will not prevent a person from falling.

4. Remove the stove controls, and move them to a safe place that you will have easy access to. Some family members have found that shutting off the kitchen circuit breaker works. In reality, I have found that this technique doesn't always work because the person with dementia may still be capable of remembering where the circuit breakers are and know how to turn them back on (especially men). If you choose to do this, have a certified electrician install a lock on the circuit breaker box.

5. If the person with dementia still cooks, install a stove sensor that will automatically shut off the stove once a person leaves the cooking area after a preset time.

6. Unplug all kitchen appliances after using them. This is a simple step to reduce the possibility that the appliance is not used correctly. A person with dementia may walk away from the unplugged appliance, believing that it is no longer working.

7. Have a smoke detector installed near the kitchen. Many companies that sell alarm systems also can install smoke detectors.

8. Know how to use the fire extinguisher in advance of a fire. Most people buy a fire extinguisher and only read the instructions when they need to use it. A crisis is not the best time to read the manual or learn how to use this device.

9. Disconnect the kitchen sink garbage disposal. If a person with dementia is doing the dishes and any utensil goes into the disposal, they will automatically retrieve it. Disable the disposal to avoid a visit to the

ER because of injury. Once the person with dementia is no longer mobile or no longer using the kitchen sink, you can easily have the wires reconnected.

Many accidents happen in the bathroom, and for the person who has moderate dementia, there are some steps that you can take to make the bathroom safer:

1. Install grab bars appropriate for the person's height in the bath or shower. Also, install grab bars on the side, next to, or in front of the toilet. A grab bar will allow the person to pull themselves up from the toilet or bathtub and give the person an added sense of well-being and independence. Grab bars can help prevent falls.

2. Place a bath seat in the shower. Many people are afraid of falling and will avoid or fight bathing for this reason. A bath seat may help to reduce bathing anxiety.

3. Install nonskid strips in the shower and on the bathroom floor. Shower mats are short and unless cleaned can have mold growing under them. Bathroom mats, because of the height change, may cause falls. Nonskid strips that you can buy at the hardware store are better. If you have tile or marble on the bathroom floor, place some nonskid strips where the person will exit the shower, around the sink, and in front of the toilet. You can also apply clear adhesive paint.

4. If the person with dementia showers by themselves and lives in a single-family home, turn down the temperature on the water heater. If they live in an apartment or condo, install an anti-scald device on the shower.

5. If the person shaves with a handheld razor, encourage them to use an electric or battery-powered razor. This will reduce facial cuts and rashes.

6. Now is the time to get rid of all bath products that are rarely used or are no longer necessary. Too many products can cause confusion. Only have items out that are to be used at the moment.

7. Install childproof locks on the bathroom cabinets. Put away everything that is not needed. Something as innocent as a cotton swab can trigger an unwanted behavior such as excessive ear cleaning that may damage an eardrum. A hairbrush can be the cause of ritualistic hair brushing. The same goes for a razor, which can trigger excessive shaving. If it is not being used at this time, put it away. An object placed out of sight is no longer a trigger for an obsessive activity.

8. Remove the door lock in the bathroom. There is no reason to have a lock on a bathroom door, especially if the person has some form of memory loss. If an explanation is needed, calmly say that the lock is broken and assure them that you will respect their privacy.

9. Change the door position. Many bathroom doors open in, not out. If the person falls, their body may block the door. For their safety, reverse the hinges on the door so that it opens outwards or if the bathroom is in the bedroom, remove the door, and put up a curtain.

10. Install a handheld shower head. This will give the person with dementia a feeling of control over their

bathing experience, especially for women who worry about wetting their hair, or for those people who are now afraid of showering.

For many people, the bedroom is their one place of comfort and security in the home. Since we spend so much time in the bedroom, it is easy for us to overlook many safety factors. As dementia progresses into the moderate phase, there are some steps that you can take to make the bedroom safer:

1. Remove the clutter. Instead of having twenty different pictures of the family on the dresser, choose four or five that are meaningful. If a person has many perfume bottles on their table, reduce the amount to two or three (and rotate the others). Clutter equals confusion for a person with dementia.

2. The same thing applies to closets. Gradually remove all clothes that are not being used. Group outfits on hangers (such as a shirt with a pair of pants or a skirt) and label them with the days of the week. This will help to reduce the person's confusion about dressing. Go through their drawers, and reduce the amount of undergarments they have. Nobody needs thirty pairs of underwear or socks. To make it easier to dress, place the undergarments that they need on the same hanger with the clothing that they will be wearing.

3. Make sure that the pathway to the bathroom is now a clear walkway. Remove anything that can block the way to the bathroom. If the person with dementia is having difficulty getting to the bathroom, this may cause them to have a premature problem with incontinence.

4. Replace the electric blanket. Moisture and electricity
    are not a safe mix. Now is the time to purchase a good
    warm blanket. Keep in mind that as a person ages
    they may need additional warmth to be comfortable
    because their skin is thinner. Check that the blanket
    can be easily laundered in your washing machine
    and does not have a care label that reads, "Dry clean
    only."

5. Remove portable space heaters. At this stage of the
    disorder space heaters are a fire hazard and the person
    who has dementia may be capable of turning up the
    heat. A high temperature on the thermostat may cause
    the person with dementia to have a difficult behavior
    or a physical problem.

6. Check the bedroom door. Because of changes in their
    personality or paranoia, many persons in the moderate
    stage of dementia will lock or barricade their door to
    insure their safety. Remove or disable the lock to allow
    you to get into the bedroom. Some people in this stage
    will move furniture to block the doorway. If you can,
    reposition the heavy furniture (such as dressers) on
    the opposite side of the room. An easy alternative is to
    have the hinges changed on the doorframe to have the
    door open out instead of in.

7. Consider replacing the nightstand. Many injuries to
    a person with dementia are caused by disorientation
    and confusion. Most accidents occur when a person
    gets out of their bed to go to the bathroom. They fall
    and hit a sharp object that injures them. Usually the
    sharp object is the nightstand. Consider replacing the
    current nightstand with one that has rounded corners.

You can also put a safe barrier around the nightstand, such as a foam pad, to soften the corners. If possible, remove the nightstand table, and replace the table light with wall sconces.

8. Place a soft mat on the floor next to the bed. If the person with dementia falls out of the bed, a thick mat may reduce injury.

9. Purchase a chiming mat to place at the side of the bed or at the bedroom door. When it sounds, it will alert you that the person is either leaving the bed or exiting the room. Many of the caregivers I work with are light sleepers; they are on constant red alert. With every toss or turn of their loved one in bed, they automatically wake up. This worry can be stopped and your sleep less interrupted if you place a chiming mat where the person with dementia normally leaves the bed, or at the front of the bedroom or bathroom door. The sound of the chime will alert you to the person's activity.

10. Install night lights, and turn them on. Place them in the bedroom, bathroom, and hallways. This may help orient a person with dementia. You should also keep in mind a person's sleeping preference. Some people like their bedroom dark. To reduce unwanted behaviors such as interrupted sleep or wandering, you may need to adjust the brightness of the lights or remove them.

Lesson Three: *Home Safety for the Person with Severe Dementia*

As the level of dementia increases, the person with dementia will need more care. Once the person is in the severe stage of dementia, there are specific things you can do to ensure their personal safety and yours.

The following are steps to take to make the kitchen safer if you have not already done so:

1. Unplug all appliances when not in use. Out of habit, a person in the severe stage may attempt to use the coffee maker, stove, or microwave. An unplugged appliance is now a nonworking or "broken" appliance. Disconnect the garbage disposal.

2. To reduce a possible accidental poisoning, remove or lock up all household cleansers. A person with severe dementia will not be able to recognize a lemon detergent from a soft drink such as lemonade, or a household cleanser that's labeled "lavender" from grape juice. They might recognize the word "lemon" or the grape color. When they were kids, these products were juice drinks. You should have poison control on the speed dial of both your home phone and your cell phone.

3. Do not reuse containers. If the container looks like or clearly states that it is oil and you put something else into it, the person with severe dementia may believe that the product is oil and use it accordingly. The same thing applies to shampoo, mouthwash, and body lotion containers.

4. Take away all items that resemble or accompany food but are not food. When a person is in the stage of severe dementia, they have lost the ability to recognize the salt shaker from the flowers. Keep mealtime and the table simple. Place on the table only the serving ware and the condiments that will be used for the

meal. If you notice that a person is over salting their food, do not put any salt on their food. Place a salt shaker with a tiny amount of salt in front of them to keep their sense of control. If they no longer need a knife to cut their food, don't put one out. Unnecessary eating utensils or items may cause confusion, anxiety, and reduced eating or socialization.

5. Avoid any foods that can cause choking hazards if eaten whole. This includes grapes, hot dogs, popcorn, or peanuts. A person with severe dementia may not chew these foods properly. You should be aware that any food if not swallowed properly may cause pneumonia or aspiration problems if the food goes down the wrong "pipe."

6. A person in the severe stage of dementia should not eat alone. Due to the possibility of not recognizing what they are eating or swallowing, there is an increased chance that they may choke on the food, vomit, or aspirate the food into their lungs.

7. Replace the glassware and china. There are many items that you can purchase that look the same as fine china and glassware but is indestructible. Using these items will reduce your stress if something is accidentally dropped. If it simply cracks, there is no glass to pick up.

8. There may come a time for some people with dementia when they may vomit during mealtimes. They may eat too much or too fast. This can be very upsetting to the family. If this occurs on more than one occasion, feed the person with dementia before the family dinner, and wash their plates and utensils separately. Keep

their plates, cups, and utensils in a separate cabinet or area. Some family members may refuse to eat off any plates in the cabinet because Grandma threw up on the plate they are now using.

9. Always check the temperature of the food before serving. Food that is too hot can burn a person's mouth; food that is too cold can be unappealing. Try to serve food at a comfortable temperature for a person with dementia. Do not serve food straight from the microwave without first checking the temperature of the plate or cup.

10. Keep in mind that food is much more than nourishment. Food means love and safety. Comfort food means home to a person with dementia. If possible, try to serve familiar meals that are comforting to them. If in doubt about what to serve, think back to what they might have said they liked in the past, or research what they might have eaten in their youth.

There are certain changes to the bedroom that will help alleviate the fear and stress of the person who has severe dementia as well as give the caregiver peace of mind:

1. Install an intercom system. It doesn't have to be an expensive or elaborate high-tech system. A baby monitor can work just as well. Place the monitor in a person's bedroom, turn the volume on, and you will be able to hear the person's actions (or non-actions) while you are in another room. A monitor will give you peace of mind while giving the person with dementia independence.

2. If you have not already done so, purchase a chiming mat. This mat will alert you that a person is leaving the bed, going to the bathroom, or leaving the bedroom.

3. If the person is incontinent or at risk for falling, buy a portable toilet. Place it near the bed, but keep in mind that the person with severe dementia might not recognize or be able to successfully use this new toilet without your help.

4. Consider replacing the current bed with a hospital bed. Because of the rails a person will be less prone to roll over and fall off the bed. Know that a hospital bed is not a restraint and should not be used for a person who wanders at night. For a person with dementia, a hospital bed can be a danger. If they are disoriented and want to get out, they may climb over the rails, which may cause a fall. Many people with dementia will slide their body down the bed and exit from the bottom (also known as scooting). A hospital bed does work well for someone with limited mobility. It also will make it easier for the caregiver to get the person in and out of bed and care for them. If your only concern is that a person may roll off the bed, purchase a bed rail that can be used on their current bed to prevent a fall, or place the bed next to a wall. When ordering a hospital bed have the prescription read for an electric three position bed- this bed will raise the leg and head area as well as raise and lower the actual bed which will make it easier for the person to get in and out of. You can lower the bed closer to the floor so if the person rolls out, there may be less injury. If the person is bed bound, this bed will make it easier on you for changing their garments and bathing them.

5. Increase the lighting in the daytime. The greater the light, the less chance of delusions or hallucinations. Increased lighting, especially if you use "bright lights," will also help reset the body's natural circadian rhythm. The person with dementia will sleep better and have fewer behavioral problems. Turn up the lights (especially in the afternoon) to reduce behavioral problems.

6. Decrease the lighting at bedtime. Studies have shown that light disrupts sleep. Some people fall asleep with the TV, then suddenly awaken, and are up for the rest of the night. The soft glow from a nightlight can cause a sleep problem when the person wakes up and sees shadows from the light. For some people, a totally dark bedroom will stop night time waking.

There will come a time where a person with dementia will have difficulty in finding or using the bathroom. Toileting problems are the number one reason for premature placement in a facility. In order to delay or avoid this situation there are some changes that you can make that will help the person with dementia use the bathroom successfully:

1. Place signs in the bedroom or hallways to point the way to the bathroom. Even in the severe stage of dementia, many people are still able to read simple signs and follow directions.

2. Paint the bathroom door a different color from the rest of the doors. Then, instead of saying, "The bathroom is the third door down the hall to the left," you can say, "The bathroom is the red door down the hall." If

you choose not to paint, you can cover the door with colorful gift wrapping paper.

3. Many of today's bathrooms are all one color. The white sink, white toilet, and white bathtub all blend into the white walls and floor. Replace the current toilet or toilet seat with one that is colorful and stands out.

4. Raise the toilet seat. There may come a time when a person who has dementia may have problems getting up from a sitting position. Instead of risking embarrassment and asking for help, many people with dementia will not want to sit down (or do the opposite: sit down for too long). You can buy raised toilet seats at a medical supply shop. Some toilet seats have arm rests that will help a person stand up and help them keep their balance.

5. Consider placing removable and washable carpet in the bathroom. Many of my clients' falls are from trying to get up from the toilet. It is better to fall on a soft carpet than a hard tiled floor.

6. Place nonskid strips in front of the toilet. Many people who have incontinence will leak or "dribble" before they make it to the toilet. A wet floor may cause a slip or fall.

7. Lock up or remove all supplies or grooming objects when not in use. When a person is in the moderate to severe stage of dementia, they may forget why they went into the bathroom in the first place. When they see a toothbrush, comb, razor, or makeup on the counter, they will become distracted. They may forget that they had to use the toilet and start grooming

themselves instead. This can cause incontinence. It will also cause an unwanted behavior in the caregiver, who now has to clean up the person with dementia and the bathroom floor.

In order to make the living room dementia friendly, there are certain changes that you can make to increase the quality of life for the person with severe dementia. Because of their memory loss, they may have difficulty recognizing familiar objects or be able to physically move around. The following are some suggestions that may help you and the person with dementia to have a better quality of life:

1. Consider buying a lift chair. This electric chair not only reclines but can also raise a person into a standing position. This will help reduce the stress on the caregiver's back from trying to help a person get up from a chair. The added benefit is that if a person falls asleep on the chair, a touch of a button turns the chair into a comfortable bed. A fabric chair is nice, but a vinyl chair is easier to clean and disinfect in case of accidents.

2. If the person's home has two levels, consider having a stair lift installed. This is an electronic seat that is on rails and takes a person up or down the stairs.

3. Remove all breakable objects. Because of the person's memory loss, many things will lose their personal value or no longer understood. Put away anything that has sentimental or monetary value.

4. Keep pathways clear. A person with dementia will have difficulty going from the kitchen to the living room, especially if there is too much furniture to

walk around. For many people, this may cause social isolation because for them it is now easier and—most importantly—safer to stay in their bedroom. Rearrange the furniture to make the living room open and inviting.

5. Above all, keep it simple. Overstimulation can cause unwanted behaviors, and so can under stimulation. Turn down or turn off the television. There are some television shows that due to their subject matter can cause aggression, disorientation, confusion, or paranoia in a person who has dementia. What a person with dementia sees on the screen is a "now" moment. They are no longer able to separate reality from fantasy. I have clients who become paranoid after watching the news. Many people who have dementia think that the person on the television is watching or talking directly to them.

Caring for a person with dementia will mean that as a caregiver you will have to make some changes in your environment. Some of these changes will be physical to ensure their safety, well-being, and quality of life. Many of the changes that I have suggested are at low or no cost. Some may be paid for by insurance or Medicare. Even if the suggestions I have given you are not paid for by insurance, the peace of mind you will have by implementing them will be worth what you have to pay. As a caregiver, your goal is to keep a person with dementia safe and comfortable where they are living now for as long as possible.

The following are some additional tips for home safety:

1. If the person smokes cigarettes, cigars, or a pipe, try to limit the time or place that they can smoke. Remove

all the ashtrays or matches, which are visual triggers; think out of sight, out of mind. If the person smokes inside the home, buy a flame retardant smoker's apron, install a smoke detector, and have a fire extinguisher handy.

2. Purchase a bathroom flood alarm that will go off if water overflows on the floor.

3. Consider buying a toilet overflow shut-off device. No matter what goes into the toilet, be it toilet paper or any other objects, once the toilet flushes and the water reaches a certain level, the toilet will automatically shut off.

4. Many people enjoy wearing socks in their homes. Apply nonskid appliqués to their socks. This will help to avoid slips and falls.

5. Check the thresholds between rooms. Thresholds will change the floor height, especially in some older homes. Anything greater than a half inch can cause a fall. If a person walks with a shuffle, a quarter-inch change in height may cause a fall.

6. Place childproof doorknob covers on all the doors to reduce wandering. If you have doorknobs that are newer and pull down to open, consider replacing them.

7. If you have a pool, install a pool fence. If you live beside a canal (or in any home that has water access), secure it. The person with dementia may at some point wander away. They may no longer be able to recognize water or may forget how to swim.

8. Disable or secure your automatic garage door. The person with dementia might realize that once pressed the garage door will go up; this will give them an opportunity to wander. They may not realize that what goes up also comes down. This is especially important in older homes that may not have the newest technology. Older homes have garage doors that will go down and keep going down no matter what. Newer homes have garage doors that will automatically stop once it senses pressure from an object or person.

9. Many older apartment buildings have elevators with doors that close quickly and automatically. Be aware that if elevator doors do not have the newer sensors installed, the person with dementia will be at risk for physical injury.

Keep in mind that a person with dementia may not always be able to verbally express their needs, wants, or feelings. But while a person who has dementia will forget what you said or what you did, they will never forget how you made them feel.

CHAPTER TEN

RESPITE CARE

As the disorder progresses, the daily hands-on care of a person who has dementia will increase. There will come a time when you will need some outside help. As much as you would like to do the care by yourself, over the long run, you can't do it alone. For a caregiver, there are no days off, no sick leave, and no vacations. Accepting that you need outside help is difficult, more difficult than you may care to admit. You have done so much for so long by yourself, and you may feel that this is *your* responsibility and yours alone. During the past few months or years—knowingly or not—you have sacrificed your life, your family, and your job.

When it comes to child care, Hillary Clinton hit the bull's eye when she said, "It takes a village to raise a child." Look around. On almost every street corner there is a day care center. In public schools, there are after-hours programs that allow children to be safe and supervised. Many large companies have on-site day care centers that will care for children from birth through age twelve. For those who can afford it, there are sleepover camps and boarding schools. Some families pay for au pairs: young people from foreign countries will come and live in homes to take care of the children; their salaries start at anywhere from $95 to $250 per week, depending on where the family lives. The au pair will clean the home, supervise the children, drop off the kids and pick them up after school, help with their homework, and take them to all of their activities (quite the deal). Some families pay for after-school sitters who will pick up their children or be waiting at home when the bus drops them off (for a small price, still a deal). And then other parents rely on family members, friends, or neighbors to care for their children until they get home (a better deal). There is also reliable bus transportation to shuttle the children to school and then to their after-school or summer activities, paid for out of taxes and run by the city parks department (the best deal). All of these options allow for young children to have supervision so that their main caregivers (the parents) can continue to work and support the family. In today's political arena, it is all about caring for the children: they have the parks, the school, after-school care, day care, summer care, and sitters. For our lawmakers and city planners, children are a soft spot.

I love children; I have two of them. But I also had parents. When my father was alive, there were few places that he could go to enjoy himself. I guess the city planners believed that older adults could and should take care of themselves. Once my father was no longer able to drive and needed to go to a doctor's appointment, shopping, or out to dinner, his options were limited to public transportation (city bus), special transportation service (STS), hiring a cab, or using me as his driver. Since he depended on others to take him where he needed to go, his choices of activities were limited. My father was legally blind. I changed and juggled my plans to work around my father's schedule. I became Dad's official driver in the family. I took him to activities, lunches, shopping, and medical appointments.

When I first started to care for my parents, I was single and working. As the years progressed, I married and had one child and six years later, another child. It was at this time in my life that my mother received a diagnosis of dementia. I then became responsible for caring for both of my parents plus my growing family. This all happened what seems like yesterday to me, but the reality is that it started over thirty years ago. I was thrust into the role of caring for my parents. I did it because I cared about them. I have two siblings who at the time lived no more than fifteen minutes away. One was married (and has been divorced for years); neither have children. They had more excuses as to why they couldn't help me or our parents than a third grader who didn't turn in their homework. At the time, there were no companion care services as there are today. Looking back, the only option for my father at the time would have been to hire a housekeeper who drove or hire a chauffeur, but my mother (who was always paranoid) didn't want strangers in the house.

I was fortunate that once my mom was diagnosed with dementia, there was a day care center in our city that was dementia-care specific and provided transportation to and from the center. Getting my father on board to send Mom to a day care center could be a chapter in itself. First, I had to convince my father that this was the best place for Mom; Once convinced that the day center would help both him and mom, dad allowed mom to go, but then it was all about how she would get there. Mom would never go on a bus so someone would have to drive her—that someone was me. I drove Mom to the day care center and back for the first three months. After a period of time, the day center bus would bring her back home. Eventually, she boarded the bus to go to the center. It took six months for Mom to be able to board the bus from our home, attend the day center, and then board the bus to bring her back home. All's well that ends well; Mom attended this center for ten years.

Unlike child care, the availability of persons or institutions to care for the elderly—especially for those who have any form of memory loss—is limited. Unless you qualify for a Medicaid grant or waiver, any assistance you will need to help you care for your loved one will have to be paid with personal funds. This means that for any inside care, such as aides, or outside care, such as a day center, the family will have to write a check unless they have good long-term care insurance.

Respite care is any form of inside care (such as aides) or outside care (such as a day center). At some point during the course of this disorder, you will need to bring in someone from the outside to help you care for the person with dementia. As much as you want to do it all, you have to be realistic and realize that you cannot handle this situation by yourself. If the goal is to allow a person to stay at home as long as possible, then the reality is that you will need to either bring someone into the home to help you or find a good local day center. If it takes a village to raise a child, it will take a village to care for a person who has dementia.

Lesson One: *The Basics of Respite Care*

Let's work with now. What do you need, what can you afford, and where do you live? These factors will determine the resources you will be able to use for care. For example, if you live in Wyoming or upstate New York, it doesn't matter how great the Medicaid payment is for a day center if the closest facility is fifty miles away. If you live in a rural area, no matter what state, even if the person with dementia qualifies, there might not be any local services to help you. Even in my county, Dade County, Florida, which has a population of over 2 million people, there are many areas that do not have dementia-specific day centers, home health workers willing to travel to certain neighborhoods, or other services. Finding a good baby sitter to care for your two-year-old triplets will be easier than finding someone to watch over an elder who has dementia.

The amount of care a person with dementia requires will change over time. As the person's daily needs change, so will the care they require, especially to handle the behavioral changes that may occur. Caring for a person who is incontinent or combative is not a job for a teenager or college student. You will have to hire a professional. Depending on where you live, this will cost you anywhere from $9 to over $25 an hour. Cost of care is based on three criteria: need, availability, and location. If you happen to live in Dade County, the current price for hourly care through an agency ranges from $12 to $25 per hour. In New York City, the price can be double or triple this amount.

The purpose of respite is to provide relief. Respite care will help you. As a caregiver, you cannot be in two places at one time, always be able or available to care for your loved one, or always want to take your loved one with you. You will need some time off from your caregiver duties and responsibilities—to spend some time either alone or with your friends and other family members. If you are ill or hospitalized, you will need outside help to take over your daily caregiver duties. This is where respite care comes in. Some families have a good support system, and the other family members will pitch in and help the main caregiver. Other families use the services of an agency to provide some relief. Day centers that are geared to a person with dementia are a great source for respite.

Keep in mind that the level of care will increase over time as the person with dementia becomes less independent and requires additional help to function independently. You may need to go through several different systems. Just like with medication, it is sometimes best to start slow. The dollar amount you can afford is an important factor. The tolerance level of the person with dementia is also something you will need to take into consideration.

Lesson Two: *Respite Options for the Person with Mild to Moderate Dementia*

The following are some potential sources of respite care.

The Housekeeper: Many people employ an outside person to help clean their house. For some, this person has become a trusted familiar fixture in your home. You feel comfortable with them, and, most importantly, so does the person with dementia. If the person with dementia is in the mild to moderate stage and is not aggressive or paranoid, your current housekeeper can be your best choice for respite care. Whether you have someone who comes in daily, twice a week, once a week, or once every two weeks, this person may be for now the ideal person to help you watch your loved one. Since your loved one at this stage will require minimal hands-on care and they already trust this person, I usually suggest hiring them for an additional day or two or five, and spread the housekeeping work over these added days. A good arrangement would be cleaning in the morning while you are present, and then having them stay with the person while you go out. Their main job while you are out is to keep an eye on the person with dementia to make sure they are safe and to be their companion.

Friends and Family: People in the mild to moderate stage of dementia will enjoy regular activities and outings. Many of my clients in these stages enjoy spending time with their friends doing activities such as playing cards, golfing, sports, shopping, and socializing with their friends and family members. Encourage these activities to keep the person with dementia active and involved. This may be uncomfortable for you, but I suggest that you tell anyone spending time with the person with dementia about the person's memory loss. It's only fair to the other people involved to understand this new situation. I have many clients who still enjoy playing golf or cards, but because of their memory problems, the others in their foursome no longer want to play with them. But in some cases, once their friends found out that the person had a form of memory loss, they continued to include them in their games and made allowances for the memory deficits. When you tell others about your loved one's memory loss, there is a risk that some people may distance or exclude your loved one from the group. Keep in mind that some people will have difficulty with dementia out of fear, lack of education about dementia, or small-mindedness. If your loved one is rejected from their usual group because of their memory loss, try not to take this rejection personally. Often friends and family may be misinformed about dementia or scared or for personal reasons are not able to deal with the situation.

When your loved one is out of the home and participating in an activity, take this time to do something that you enjoy or do a task that you have put off. Use this time to pay the bills, grocery shop, or do any of the things that you would normally do but while your loved one is with you would usually take two or three times longer.

High School and College Students: Students are a terrific resource. High school students need to have volunteer hours. For a person in the mild stage of dementia, a student will provide a human connection and a link to a younger generation. A person in the mild stage of dementia has a lot of knowledge and love to share. Many high school students are missing this connection and guidance from their elders, who may no longer be alive or who live far away. Pairing these two age groups together at this stage is often a good fit. They can both learn and share with each other. An added benefit is that it may fill a missing void in both of their lives. Many families no longer live close together; the high school student can become a surrogate grandchild. From one generation to another, through this student, the elder can share relationship, knowledge, and life experiences with another person. They can tell each other stories, give and get advice, and have adventures together. If your loved one enjoys or once enjoyed playing tennis, baseball, or golf or liked fishing, cooking, gardening, knitting, discussing philosophy or current events, try to find a student who has similar interests. This will help your loved one remain active in life. You can also check with your local church or temple to see if they have students who would like to help or need volunteer hours.

College students, especially those who are studying to be a doctor or nurse (or anyone in the health care field), are often a good choice to provide respite care. Because of their workloads at school, many students cannot manage a full-time job and will welcome or need the extra money that you will give them. For many of my caregiver clients who have a spare room in their home, I have suggested that they barter the room for care. This has worked out well for many families. The student needs a place to live, and you need someone to relieve you so that you can do what you need to do. This situation can be a win-win arrangement.

Be aware that no matter who the boarder is, you should draw up a contract. This is especially important if the person is in college or for any individual with whom you are bartering services. Spell out specifically what is allowable and what you will not tolerate. Include what places in the house are for their use and the times of use. For example, put in writing the times that the pool, hot tub, or sauna will be available for their use as well as who can use them and the specific number of people allowed in your home or on your property at any given time. With common areas, such as the kitchen and living room, make the use and time clear. Include in this contract the house rules regarding smoking, drinking, drugs, certain foods, dietary customs, having friends over, pets, and curfew hours, to name a few situations that may arise. Be honest with yourself as to what you can and cannot tolerate. Respect yourself and your wishes as a caregiver. Above all, always remember that it is your home. Do not ever feel that because you now need or like a certain person, you will allow inappropriate or uncomfortable behavior.

Of special note is that no matter what your situation is, review your homeowners insurance policy to determine your liability. Make sure that you understand the current coverage, and change or update your policy to include this additional person. Accidents happen. Find out what you, as a homeowner, will be responsible for. Before hiring or bringing in anyone into your home, use common sense, and do a background check. Most people interested in this kind of arrangement will be good, but there are always exceptions. They may look good on paper or during an interview, but they can have emotional or mental baggage you might not want to handle. Be smart. Do an internet search on the person's name, and hire a company that can do a thorough background check. If you are using an agency, make sure that the agency does a thorough background check. This should include checking all states. People reinvent themselves when they move to another place. Protect yourself and your family. Do not ignore your gut reaction. If you feel something might be wrong, it probably is. Have a termination clause in your agreement.

Neighbors: There was a time, up until not so long ago where two, three, or four generations of families lived under one roof or on the same block. Back then, everyone knew everybody and each neighborhood was a family. Okay, maybe one large dysfunctional family, but a family. No matter what, everybody in the neighborhood looked out for one another. Flash forward to today. In today's fast paced world it seems like everyone is moving in or moving out. If you look closely, there are still many communities that have a family feel—you just need to reach out. I have several clients who were only happy to check in with or help care for their neighbor who has memory loss, if they were asked. It's the neighborly thing to do. They will look out their window or listen to the sound of the elevator and the key in the door to know that their neighbor is home. Approach them and ask them if they would be able and willing to check in on your loved one, help them with meals, transportation, medication, or stay with them when you need to go out. Offer to pay them for their help. Some may be offended by your good intentions of paying them, but others may welcome the opportunity to have additional income. If the neighbor refuses money, give them prepaid gift cards at local stores or restaurants, in a handwritten card where you appreciate them for their caring.

Lesson Three: *Working with Agencies*

Some agencies in your area may provide companionship service. I call this service "rent a friend" or "rent a family member." In the beginning stage of dementia, your loved one may only need a person who will monitor their medications or go with them to a ball game or a doctor's appointment, especially if you live out of town. If the person enjoys fishing or swimming, this type of agency will provide companionship and will accompany your loved ones to the outings that they enjoy. Know that even if the aide has been trained in dementia -it doesn't mean that they understood all the training or that the trainer was good; it just means that they have a certificate that says they took a one or four-hour course on dementia. I know many caregivers who have successfully used this type of agency. Companions will go with the person with dementia to the casino, hair salon, shopping, lunches, movies, theater, religious activities, etc. The caregiver dresses normally (not in a uniform). They watch over the person with dementia and accompany them to their events and activities. The companion will also help clean and organize the home. Paid companions can help the person get in or out of the bathtub, prepare meals, lay out clothing, remind them of medication, and help pay their bills. What some of these agencies will not provide is hands-on care. The companions cannot legally bathe, feed, give medication, or change their diaper. For this you will need to consider hiring a person from a different type of agency. Check to see if the person who is hired is able to give medication.

Using a paid companion agency during the mild or moderate stage of dementia can help the person with dementia remain independent for as long as possible. When I first was introduced to this form of care seven years ago, I was wary and cynical. I spent a lot of time researching, and I found that many of these companies are worth what you have to pay for their services. Companion agencies allow the person in the mild to moderate stage of dementia (who does not yet need hands-on care) to continue living an independent life. This in itself is invaluable. Using this type of agency will give you the peace of mind knowing that your loved one is being cared for and attending activities that they enjoy. It also has an additional benefit in that you and your loved one will not have to change their current lifestyles. Everybody benefits.

As the dementia progresses, the persons care needs will change. The person with dementia will require more hands-on care in their activities of daily living (ADLs) such as feeding, toileting, grooming, walking, and transferring. In addition, their independent activities of daily living (IADLs), such as using appliances, paying bills, taking medication, cooking, and going to the doctor, will require more assistance from you. As the disorder progresses, you may need to go outside of your immediate family or current respite provider to manage the increasing needs of the person with dementia. You will need to reevaluate the care as the dementia progresses. What works well today might not work tomorrow for you or the person with dementia. Overtime you may need to add or change services or caregivers. Many of the families I work with use a mixture of services.

A full-service care agency should be a state approved home health care agency. They have home health aides (HHA), certified nursing assistants (CNA), licensed practical nurses (LPN), and registered nurses (RN) on their staff. The cost will increase according to the care needed. A HHA and CNA are capable of providing for daily needs such as grooming, feeding, bathing, transferring and driving. As the dementia progresses, you may need a person, who is qualified to provide additional care such as medication which a CNA can do. Once a person needs skilled care such as wound management or tube feedings you may need a RN. Many of my families have a full time HHA or CNA and then hire a RN to come in for some care. Others may have a good CNA that can provide for all care. The care that is needed will depend on the situation.

Some agencies employ people who want to work for only a few hours a day; others have people who want to work daily, and there are those who want to live in the person's home. Find out in advance what type of agency you are hiring and the amount of care they can provide. This is really important, especially in the middle to end stage of dementia, when stability and consistency are crucial.

Another important aspect is cost of care. Prices will vary where you live and for many of us we may feel that the price is either a bargain or set in stone. Don't be fooled. Since my clients live in South Florida and the children live in different states, they know what it costs in their state for care—and think that this is the going rate. Wrong thinking! Call different agencies in the area that your loved one lives in, ask about the rate and negotiate. In South Florida the rate varies from $125.00 to $400.00 per day for a live in aide depending on the agency. If a person has long term care insurance, the insurance company may give you a list of agencies that they use and so you are lead to believe that they are the best or only agencies. You need to know that many of these agencies have or had a contract with the insurance policy, and at one time accepted the daily rate—they may no longer do so. It will now cost you more out of pocket if you go with that agency. If you live in Vermont, New York, or Las Vegas and the going rate for an aide is $40.00 an hour, when you hear from an agency or a friend where your loved one lives the rate is $25.00 per hour, this may sound like a great deal. The reality is that the going rate is actually $14.00 per hour or less—you are overpaying.

When it comes to private duty aides who work out of an agency, know that even though they have been referred by a friend, family, or hospital—they may be overcharging you. Before I was hired by the family as a geriatric care manager, this family was paying the private duty aide $400.00 per day to live in. The family assumed that based on where they lived and the referral this was the normal cost. At first they were price conscious with my fee. I went in, assessed the situation, made recommendations, and suggested other agencies that they should contact. They loved the new aide I placed for

$125.00 per day. The family went from $2,800.00 per week to $975.00 per week. By using my services, I saved the family $1,825.00 per week or $5,300.00 per month. The reality is that I saved this family $54,600.00 a year.

Once a person bonds to a hired caregiver, and they are a good fit with your family, you will want to make sure that they can continue to provide the care needed in the long term. They might need additional training to understand and deal with a person who has dementia. As a caregiver, you will have to be flexible. If the person can only work days and you are "in love" with the aide, then you might consider hiring another person at night. This will cost more: additional night care or split shifts will double or triple the cost of care. I recommend that you find someone who can stay with the person full-time. Finding a full-time aide is not easy. You might have to go through several caregivers and agencies until you find the right fit. As difficult as this process is, even as you may go through what seems like a revolving door of caregivers, you will find someone who is right for the person with dementia and for your family. When you do find this person (and trust me, you will eventually), all that you went through will be well worth it.

Lesson Four: *How to Find and Hire the Right Caregiver*

When calling an agency, be realistic and honest about your needs. This is not the time to beat around the bush to get just any breathing person into your home to take care of your loved one. As desperate as you may be to have relief, you will need to tell the agency what your current needs are (especially when the person with dementia is living with you), and your family situation. I found this out the hard way. Over the past years my mother's dementia changed and so did her needs. I have two large dogs and two cats. I also have kids. The agency sent me some wonderful and some not so wonderful people who either were terrified of dogs, were allergic to cats, or didn't know how to deal with dementia. I spent many days, nights, and weekends locking up the animals or keeping them out of the common rooms. If the person walked outside to do laundry or take out the trash, the dogs would attack the door and bark like crazy. For years, I was beyond stressed—I was a nervous wreck. My days at work were stressful enough without having to worry about whether the person who was caring for my mother was encountering my four-footed family members. It took me years before I finally broke down and told the current agency (I had gone through several at this point) that they could only send me someone who could deal with cats and large dogs, and that my mother had, at that point, end-stage dementia and would need real hands-on help.

When I became honest about my family situation, the agency sent Lucille. I like to believe that every agency has one person they send out for special cases. This agency had Lucille. Think of the best nanny you could possibly imagine and then multiply her by 12. Lucille came in and took in our situation, and nothing fazed her. She took control of my mother, the animals, and my children who were now teenagers. She also took control of me. With her strength and guidance, Lucille transformed my chaotic home into one that is calm and spiritual. Lucille also puts up with my daily stupidity. She has become my best friend and mentor. The care she gives my mother is unbelievable. With over five years of being bed-bound, my mother never had a bed sore and was so well-fed and taken care of that she was discharged (kicked out of) hospice twice. If not for Lucille caring for my family, and for me, this book would not have been finished. Without Lucille, I would no longer be working, but I would still be around; you could find me in the psychiatric ward at my hospital. Without proper back up, providing full-time care for a person with dementia can cause a breakdown.

Thoroughly screen anyone who is coming into your home. Your home is your safety zone. There are many honest persons out there, but then there are those people who only *look* good when you first meet them or on paper. Know that many references are bogus. In the caregiving field, a reference is only as good as the person who is giving it. Many people are afraid of giving a bad reference. I used to be but no longer am one of those people. Over the past sixteen years I have gone through several agencies and many aides. I still remember one particular aide because she was beyond inept. She actually fled my house and left the back door open (when my mother was still mobile) because she didn't feel safe. My house has a pool, and since the kids were older (they were then nine and fifteen years old), it never occurred to me to fence it in. I was lucky to be home when this situation happened. In my home, I have a monitored alarm system and large dogs. (Did I mention that one of my dogs is a German shepherd?) My house is beyond safe! After fleeing my home with the back door wide opened at 7:30 at night, the aide later used me as a reference. There was no way I was going to help her work with another family. I checked through other sources later and found out that she had worked for several other agencies and left their homes the same way she left mine. At the time I hired her, she was not working through an agency but came "highly recommended." This person later contacted me and wanted to work for me again. If she was the only choice, I would quit my job and change my mother's diapers myself (I would find a good therapist to help me get over my PTDD) before I allowed her back into my home.

Ask the agency if the person is properly trained in dealing with dementia. Caring for a person who has dementia will mean understanding the daily changes in their memory, which will affect their care. A person who has been properly trained in dementia care (such as taking educational courses and reading books) will have a better understanding of the care that is needed. It doesn't mean that they will be the best person; it just means that they might have better insight. Some people, no matter what their training is, still will be useless. As my dad often said, "You can't make a silk purse out of a sow's ear."

Check with the agency to be sure the person who is hired is insured and bonded. Find out if the agency is their employer or just a referral source. If the agency is an employer, they will handle all of the responsibilities of taxes and Social Security. Since the agency is responsible for scheduling, if the aide is sick and cannot show up for work, the agency should send out a replacement. Many employer agencies include benefits for their employees, such as health insurance and workers' compensation. This is why they charge a higher fee.

If the agency is a referral source, the aide you now have working for you may be an independent contractor. You pay them directly. Find out in advance what will happen if the aide gets a better job or full-time job somewhere else. Will the agency replace them? As a caregiver who depends on outside care, you cannot afford to be without back up.

Find out if the agency is available for contracting twenty-four hours a day, seven days a week. Many agencies operate from 9 AM to 5 PM. I learned this lesson the hard way. An agency that I normally used and trusted should have sent the relief aide on Christmas Day. The aide never showed up, and when I called, all I got was an answering machine. They called me back Monday morning to apologize. On New Year's weekend, after several phone calls placed during the week, I heard back from the agency on Friday afternoon. The manager of the agency assured me that she was sending a reliable person to relieve Lucille. By Friday night, since no one had called me back to confirm the weekend relief aide, it was apparent that the agency didn't have anyone for me. I called the agency back and got a machine. I was at my wits' end, and so was Lucille, who needed time off to be with her family.

As a last-ditch resort, I opened up my personal files and placed phone calls to three of the people on my team. Within the hour, they called me back with the names of agencies they use, and I put in calls to them. Picture this moment: it's after eight o'clock on the Friday of New Year's weekend, and by now Lucille and I have devised a plan (actually it was the same plan we used for Christmas, when she cared for Mom and then I took over until she returned the next day). Both of us would need to juggle our plans, and maybe our Plan B wasn't the best for either of us, but it was a plan. As God or providence would have it, within the hour all three agencies called me back. Directors of two of the agencies offered to come and stay in my home, and the third agency representative said that they could have someone in place by New Year's Eve. Lucille and I decided to stay with our Plan B. Since then, I have had the opportunity to meet with all of these agencies, and I know I can count on them to give my clients superior service.

If the person you are caring for lives alone, you might need a different type of caregiver than if they live with you or your family. Be realistic about what you want to handle or can handle and what will be the responsibilities of the person you hire. During the first several years of caring for my mother, I made all of her meals except for lunch during the week, which was served at the day center. Breakfast was easy for me since I was already up and needed to feed my kids. The same went for dinner. For many years, I had a caregiver who was great at giving Mom her bath, but she was a disaster in the kitchen. If the person is living alone when you hire an aide, I suggest that you also hire a geriatric care manger to do an unannounced home visit on a weekly basis to assess the situation, coordinate doctor's appointments, and give recommendations for daily activities. The geriatric care manager will be a valuable resource and will keep you up to date as to what is happening in the home.

As the years have progressed (and through many different caregivers) I have met some wonderful people, as well as others whom I wasn't so thrilled with. And then there were those caregivers who made my days and nights a living nightmare. Any day you want to trade some horror stories, just contact me. After sixteen years of being Mom's sole caregiver, I have experienced almost everything you can imagine. I had one aide who was doing the laundry in my house for her entire neighborhood, another who spent hours on her knees praying, one who told me unless I had certain cable channels she was quitting, and another who requested home delivery of a certain publication. I have had people who asked for or just took any portable appliances they wanted—grills, bread makers, toaster ovens, coffee makers, rotisseries. I would make weekly trips to Costco and five trips to Publix, and still there was nothing left to eat in the house. Food, detergent, paper towels, and toilet paper just "magically" disappeared. Forget about the dry goods. A five-pound bag of rice—gone. Laundry detergent, dishwashing soap, canned vegetables, and anything that came in a jar—gone. I have had to purchase (or should I say repurchase) over the years several sets of flatware, plates, drinking glasses, dish towels, and more cooking utensils than you can imagine.

The same goes for pots, pans, and knives. I have a weakness for good cookware. As a caregiver, in order to maintain your sanity, there are certain things you will need to keep constant. For me, my sanity is good cooking equipment. After noticing that either all of my utensils or my supplies were missing or being totally destroyed by the aides, I would go out to the store and buy replacements. Some I would put in my kitchen, and others I bought and stored at a friend's house. I will never forget the day when Lucille (who loves to cook) went from weekend relief to full-time, and she questioned the condition of the current cooking ware. Once I got to know Lucille, I went to my friend's home and brought over all the new pots and pans I had stored in her home. Lucille and I share a love of the Food Network and really good cookware. When I bought a replacement set of professional knives, by Lucille's reaction, you would have thought she had won the lottery when she saw the knife set. But I felt I had won the lottery because I knew that Lucille would take good care of my possessions.

You are the boss. This is an employer-employee relationship. Talk about what you want and expect them to do. Be direct and tell the aide what she is required to do. Be clear in what you want and state what you want. Aides are not mind readers. Schedule a weekly meeting. This will give both you and the aide an opportunity to discuss the care plan and have an open communication so that you both can share in the care and make adjustments. Knowing that you will have this meeting will allow for an exchange of observations and suggestions and it is the time to bring up issues that might me difficult.

Keep in mind that this is your home. The person who you are bringing in will have access to important documents such as Medicare, social security, and banking information. If you have valuables, such as jewelry, art work or fine china pieces; insure, secure or remove them.

The reason I am sharing this with you is because, as a caregiver, you should know that you are vulnerable. Years ago, I was like many of you: desperate to have someone stay in my home and help care for my loved one. Because a person is sent from an agency, we tend to believe that they are skilled. Many aides and agencies may take advantage of your lack of knowledge. When I first started to care for Mom, I didn't know what to do or what to expect. As a new caregiver, I wasn't informed. There were no books on the market like this one to help me understand or navigate the ins and outs of hiring a person to work in my home. I believed the agency would send the best person to care for my mother when I was not home and even when I was home. Even though I was an expert in dementia care, at that time, I knew nothing about hiring in help or working with agencies. Over the years I had hired I had hired in nanny's and housekeepers- but dealing with a person to care for my parents was different. I now know what to do and what is expected. As a caregiver, you now will know too.

Through the years, I have had paid caregivers who asked either me or my children to help them turn Mom in her bed or to help them change her diaper. Some of their cooking skills left much to be desired, and it became my responsibility, after working all day, to make Mom's meals. I have had aides who cooked meals for themselves and left it up to me to cook for and feed Mom. I have had aides who knew that I would be at home on Sunday and would take advantage of me and my easygoing nature by asking for an hour off and then disappearing for several hours. Call me naïve; call me stupid; call me human. As a caregiver, if I was staying home that day anyway, at the time I didn't see any harm in a person taking some time off for herself. I was so desperate to have someone care for my mom that I was willing to put up with and tolerate any behavior. I had no knowledge of other choices.

Years ago, when I started to care for my parents, my options were limited to what was then available. That was then; this is now. After spending years working in the field of dementia, dealing with aides and agencies both personally and professionally, I now know how home health agencies work. I know what the person you hire is responsible for, and I can sum it up in two words: total care. Any aide you hire is responsible for the care of your loved one. Aside from the daily care that is needed, such as bathing, feeding, transferring, and toileting, care also includes cooking, laundry, and cleaning the area that the person lives in. Light housekeeping is a part of their job. Depending on the agency, grocery shopping and taking your loved one to medical appointments may and should be included in an aide's duty.

If you hire a private aide who comes highly recommended, be sure to check out the local prices. I have had clients who paid a very high price for an aide's services, not knowing that they were being overcharged.

When I say that a caregiver is vulnerable, I mean that to continue living your life—with your family, your job, your social activities—you will be dependent on outside help. At times you may be desperate. There are many good people out there, but be aware that some people will take advantage of your good nature and naïveté. As caregivers, we are often desperate. Because we are desperate, naïve, or stressed, there may be times when we will accept or tolerate anyone in our home and give into any demands they make because we believe that we need this person to help care for our loved one. Do not be discouraged or feel that you have no choice but to keep employing a person even if they drain you financially, physically, or emotionally. Finding a good caregiver is a lot like dating. You have to kiss a few toads until you find your prince. The first kiss can be deceiving; if you feel that the person is not working out, let them go.

Lesson Five: *Keeping the Person with Dementia Active and Engaged*

To get through this disorder, you will need to be realistic, informed, and educated. The care that is needed will depend on the person's memory loss, but you also have to take into account their physical and emotional well-being. Many of my first-time clients leave the doctor's office devastated because the doctor tells them or the family that they have mild cognitive impairment (MCI) or mild dementia. Despite what you may think, a diagnosis of MCI or mild dementia is not the end of the world. Many people never progress beyond this stage. The person is still able to maintain their current life and remain active in the community. Below I have listed some suggestions for keeping a person with MCI or mild dementia as active and engaged as possible. The goal is to keep them active and engaged because stimulation helps the brain stay involved. Stagnation will cause a decline, and so will depression and stress.

1. Contact local colleges and universities. Many of them have classes or seminars for seniors at low or no cost that will help with mental stimulation.

2. Check with your local religious organization or congregation. They need people who are able to volunteer to do much needed work, such as mailings, phone calls, or being a greeter. They may also have

classes like art or religious studies that may be of interest.

3. Look to the malls. Many now have mall-walker clubs. They also may have arts and crafts businesses where people can paint plates or objects that will become keepsakes (or personalized holiday gifts) for the family, or check out readings at a bookstore.

4. Call your local senior center. Many of them have art, music, current events, or exercise classes that might appeal to your loved one.

5. Check the newspapers for listings of upcoming and ongoing local events that might be of interest. Some have personal sections that can pair your loved one with a new person who enjoys their current activities.

6. Consider hiring a local professional. I have clients who really enjoy and can do what they love as long as they are properly supervised. Many of my clients enjoy the outdoors: deep-sea fishing, golf, tennis, hunting, swimming, or shopping. Take your loved one's needs, limitations, and capabilities into consideration. Be honest with the people who will be working with them.

As the disorder progresses, your loved one will need additional help to keep active. Some people with dementia fall into the "tweeny" stage. A tweeny is when a person is between two stages. The person with dementia is no longer capable of doing some things on their own and will need some help, but they are capable of doing other things by themselves. This might be for you (and the person with dementia) the hardest stage because it makes care difficult to figure out. The person with memory loss now needs some help, but will fight you for their personal independence. When in this stage, a person with dementia will still look the same but they will have moments when they will lose their capacity to reason, use logic, or be able to consider consequences for their actions or inaction. A person with dementia will live in two worlds. As a caregiver, so will you. At one moment the person with dementia will have clarity, and in the next moment they may experience confusion. It is just as confusing and frustrating for them as it is for you. The key to successfully deal with this stage is that you'll need to realize and recognize that each day, hour, or minute is a new moment for them.

The following are a few suggestions for helping a person in the "tweeny" stage of mild to moderate dementia stay engaged:

1. Go with them to activities. Keep them active in things they enjoy. If possible, bring them with you to activities you enjoy.

2. Invite friends over. Explain what is going on in advance. You need human contact, and so does the person with dementia.

3. Check the local paper for upcoming events. Find something that looks fun and interesting for you and your loved one. Before you go, realize that the person with dementia, having initially said yes to an outing, may change their mind when they get there and want to go back to the safety and familiarity of their home. Plan in advance that you may have to leave before the event starts or ends.

4. Encourage family members to either visit with or take out a person who has dementia. Something as simple as a ride in a car, going to a movie, running errands, or a drive through a fast food restaurant can be a pleasure to a person who has dementia.

5. Look for government resources. Medicare will pay for a short time for physical, occupational, and speech therapy. The time the therapist spends in your home will benefit both the person with dementia and you.

6. Take the person to religious services. Some people will enjoy attending religious services even though they may have not done so in years.

7. Play music. Music therapy has been shown to unlock past memories and to calm an agitated person as well as to motivate a person with memory problems. Play music that they liked. Familiar music from their teenage years through early adulthood works well.

8. Watch movies and television shows that are in black and white. Most people will enjoy watching episodes of *I Love Lucy*, *The Honeymooners*, and *Hogan's Heroes*, etc. The shows are from a time in the past that they may connect too—they are short and funny and have few characters to follow. Black-and-white shows are easier to follow than color. You can rent these shows to play in your home, or they may be available through your local cable channel.

Lesson Six: *How to Evaluate Adult Day Centers*

As memory loss progresses and the person is in the moderate to the early severe stage of dementia, the most valuable and cost-effective solution may be to enroll them in a local adult day care center. Day centers provide a safe environment and have activities that are specifically designed for a person with memory loss. I refer to this form of respite as "out care."

Walking through the mall or going to the grocery store, although it is an outing, may not be a sufficient activity to stimulate a person with dementia, depending on their stage. They may need more to keep them engaged in order to maintain their dignity and independence. They also need structure and socialization. This is where a day center comes in. A day center, especially a good center, will allow for the six S factors. These factors are the most important things you can do for a person with dementia. A good day center should provide daily stimulation, socialization, success, self-actualization, structure, and security. A good day center will provide all six. Where you live will determine which center your loved one can attend. (Some rural and urban communities' nearest dementia day centers may be miles and hours away, making it impractical or impossible for your loved one to attend.)

Everybody needs to be stimulated. If you do not use it, you lose it. Color, shapes, and sounds keep us active participants in our life. As humans, we are social beings. We need people in our life to talk to, exchange thoughts or ideas with, or just converse with. We also need to be physically touched by others. This is how we connect. When you succeed at something, you feel good about yourself, and this feeling stays with you and carries over into areas of your life. Self-actualization is being able to meet your full potential. Structure allows a person to know what is going to happen and what is expected of them. Security is physical and emotional comfort. There is also a seventh S: self-determination. This is where people are free to make their own choices. A good day center will have a choice of ongoing activities which allows them the freedom to choose the activities that they would like to participate in. A good day center will increase the quality of life for the person with dementia and for you the caregiver.

My mother's experience at a day center and the experiences of hundreds of my clients who have used these centers testify to the benefits for both the person with memory loss and the caregiver. The stimulation and socialization a center can provide will make everyone's life better. When choosing a day center here are some of the things you should look for:

1. Cleanliness. A good day center will be clean and bright. People may have incontinence, but they will be quickly cleaned and changed into dry clothing. You want a bright facility. Dark environments will not only be uninviting but also be depressing and may cause behavior problems.

2. Staffing. Ask about the number of staff and the training the staff has as well as the total number of people they are caring for. Be realistic. One caregiver can only watch or take care of three or four people at one time. Depending on the care your loved one needs or the care you feel comfortable with, consider sending an aide to give the personal care your loved one may need (if your finances will allow it).

3. Activities. Check the current schedule. At first, choose the days with scheduled activities that you think your loved one will enjoy. Realize that a person who has dementia may get great pleasure from an activity you never knew of (or considered) or one they found enjoyable or interesting in the past. Remember that because structure is important for a person who has dementia, plan on the person attending a day center

three to five days a week. Going less often may cause confusion.

4. Gender balance. Some centers have more men on certain days. If your loved one is a man, ask the center which days will be best for them to attend.

5. Safety. A person who has dementia has a good chance of wandering away from the center. They may at some point get bored, lose interest in the activity, or want to go home. Make sure that the center has some controls in place so that a person who has dementia cannot leave the grounds.

6. Choices. Everybody needs a choice. Try to find a center that has two or more ongoing activities at one time. A person with dementia may not want to do an arts and craft project and may prefer some physical exercise or down time. Being forced into an activity that's not enjoyable may cause a difficult behavior or their refusal to attend.

7. Language. We live in a multicultural word, and many people are bilingual. As the disease progresses, a person whose second language is English will begin to lose the second language and revert to their first language. Try to find a center that has clients with similar languages.

8. Range of activities. Activities should be tailored to the level and ability of the person with dementia. A high-functioning person will be bored with an activity that is below their level of capability, and a low-functioning person will be frustrated with an activity that is beyond

their capability. Either of these situations may cause a difficult behavior.

9. Quiet time. During the day, there will be times when a person with dementia will need some "down time" and have moments when they need to rest, reflect, or just get away from too much stimulation. A good day center will have a calm, quite area for a person with dementia to relax, unwind, and recharge themselves.

10. Hours. Check that the hours of operation fit your needs as a caregiver and your schedule. You will also have to factor in the schedule of your loved one. If they are a morning person, going to a day center may be easy. If they prefer to sleep in or lack motivation, attending a day center will be a challenge.

Lesson Seven: *Finding a Support Group*

Another form of respite that often gets overlooked is support groups. Support groups are a terrific opportunity to meet other people who are going through a similar situation and to learn how they are handling it. I like to think of these groups as "safety in numbers" because it helps to know that you are not alone. After running a group for several years for the Alzheimer's Association and attending many other groups as a guest speaker, I've learned that there are many different types of groups and that it's important to find a group you feel comfortable in. You may have to try out several different groups before you find one that clicks for you. Some groups are more geared to spouses, others to children. Some groups have a higher number of men than women, or vice versa. I have found that even though the main issue is the same, the way caregivers approach and deal with dementia will be different because the needs of a spouse will be different from the needs of a child. I've also noticed that the more women in a group, the quieter the men become—which may be why fewer men come to support groups.

Support groups can be a terrific form of respite because they give you a "real" reason to get out of the house. Most groups meet once a month for about an hour and a half, although times may vary, and some groups (like mine) meet for two or three hours. I have clients who attend four different meetings a month. The good thing about a support group is that it provides a safe environment to discuss what's going on in your life. Our friends and family members, although well-meaning, may not always be the best source of information and ideas. There are times when we may not want to share with family or friends, or they may be tired of listening to our complaints. Sometimes it's better to unload around sympathetic listeners. Another benefit of support groups is that participation is up to you. You can share as little or as much as you want to. I have found that as time goes on, the quietest person in the group becomes one of the best participants.

In order to find a support group that meets your needs, contact your local Alzheimer's Association, or check with your local hospital. If there are no groups in your area, consider starting your own. Place an ad in the local paper, or check with your place of worship. It also helps to ask a professional social worker who has experience running groups and is knowledgeable about dementia to lead the group.

Lesson Eight: *Consider Alternative Care*

There may come a time when the care you provide in the home is no longer enough. Your loved one is now having problems that make it difficult to manage their care even with an aide.

Nobody wants to talk about or consider placing their loved one in a continuing care retirement community (CCRC), an independent living facility (ILF), an assisted living facility (ALF), or a nursing home, but there will come a time, despite your best efforts, when this may be your best or only choice.

In the beginning, a CCRC may be a good choice for care. These communities offer a range of support, from independent living through end-of-life care, all on the same campus. The ones I have visited are more like a four-star hotel or a cruise ship. They have every amenity you might want: concierge services, gourmet restaurants, gym, spa, and golf course. Forget about the luxury, which is unbelievable; the most important thing they provide is health care for life. If your loved one doesn't have a current long-term care insurance plan, moving your loved one into a CCRC may be your best long-term financial bet. Once you pay the up-front fee and monthly maintenance charge, you and they are financially better off. No matter what the care needed, all future care is covered by the monthly fee.

If something sounds too good to be true, you need to do your research. Check the refund policy in case the person hates the place and wants to move out. No matter how terrific the place looks, you need to verify their license, check their rating and financial solvency, and look at accreditation. A CCRC is a lifelong care choice. When a person needs to change from their current residence, are they able to move easily from one area of care to another? You should visit all of the facility's care areas (even those you may not need or think that you will need) before signing the contract. Ask about rate increases and current occupancy rates. Ask how they determine a move from the current living area. You are spending a lot of money for a life care facility; you need to learn as much as possible about it. Each CCRC will offer different services and products. You will have to do some legwork to find out which facility will be better for you and your loved one. Some continuing care retirement communities do not require hefty up-front fees. There are some campuses where you pay as you go through their different levels of care.

When the time comes that your loved ones need additional care and safety, the first place you should look into is an independent living facility (ILF). An ILF is like living in your own apartment—but with benefits. Many of these facilities have an on-site restaurant that provides one or two meals a day. The apartments have full kitchens, and residents can come and go as they please. They also provide transportation to doctors, banking, and shopping. Many offer scheduled activities to keep the residents active and engaged. Most have after-dinner programs and outings to local venues such as movies, plays, and community outings. If a person needs minimal care and you want to help them maintain their quality of life, an ILF is a good place to start. It's like living in a condominium with benefits. When the time comes that they need some additional assistance, you can hire an aide, and for the time being, they will be able to remain where they are.

There will come a time when the person will need additional care. This is where an assisted living facility (ALF) comes in. An ALF is for a person who is still independent but needs some additional help with their bathing, grooming, toileting, and transferring. A good ALF will have a choice of daily activities and provide all meals, transportation, housekeeping, and assistance with medication and medical appointments. They should also provide for the daily care your loved one needs. Depending on the care needed, the price will vary—many have a sliding scale. Read the contract carefully. If the person is in the early stage of dementia, visit their dementia ward. If the ALF doesn't have a dementia-specific floor for their care, ask and get in writing what their transfer plan is. As a caregiver, you don't want to find out at the last minute that Mom is going to be transferred to another facility that you haven't already checked out.

A high price doesn't guarantee the best care. Whether you have chosen a small, family-owned establishment or a top-of-the-line corporate care facility, the person who owns or runs the facility may change, and so might the care. Verify the license, check out their rating, look at accreditation, and check with a local long-term care ombudsman. Before you sign any contract, have an attorney review it. I have known several people who fell in love with all the amenities and didn't ask the serious questions, like what happens if Mom becomes difficult or the care that she needs over time changes. Some of my clients moved in only to find out a month later that this was not an appropriate place based on the level of care they actually needed. A facility may sign someone up just to get them in the door, only to slam them later with higher prices. A contract is a legal document that spells out obligations. Many of the amenities featured in their brochures might not be covered, such as laundry service, incontinence products, and meals delivered to the room. I know that this sounds like a lot to check into, but it's better to be prepared. This is going to be one of the toughest decisions that you will make.

As the person with dementia declines, they may need to be placed in a nursing home that will provide around-the-clock care. Fewer than twenty of my clients have been placed in a nursing home. A nursing home is for individuals who have medical conditions that need constant observation or for those in the end stage of dementia who are no longer able to walk, communicate, participate, or eat even with assistance. For the past five years, my mom would have been a candidate for a nursing home, but because I cared for her at home and did not place her in a facility her long-term care policy wouldn't cover her care. For some families, they may choose to place their loved one in a nursing home in order to receive the insurance benefits. I check out nursing homes frequently. Take it from me: they are not the happiest places on the planet, but they will provide the health care that a person needs. A nursing home will not replace the individual attention that a person can get at home. The facilities staff are often overworked and underpaid. If Mom needs to have her diaper changed at 2 AM, it might not happen at that time, and she will have to wait till the next shift to be cleaned. I've spoken with many aides over the years about the care they give in nursing homes. In a nutshell, the aides reported to me that they are overworked, underpaid, unappreciated, and understaffed. Once a person is placed in a nursing home, you should consider hiring outside help so that your loved one is cared for properly. There are some nursing homes that are terrific and give great care. Due to my clients, I often visit different facilities. During the week days many are filled with staff and activities, however on weekends, the staff and activities are reduced. As a caregiver you will need to check out local as well as distant nursing homes to find a place that you feel comfortable with.

CHAPTER ELEVEN

SAVING YOUR SANITY

This chapter is going to tackle some of the concerns brought up by many caregivers from my support groups and many of my clients as well as my personal thoughts and feelings. Read through them all. Certain things may apply to you now, others may affect you later, and some might be good information to pass on to others. I have included some situations in this chapter because I heard through the years from caregivers that if they "take [fill in the blank] away," their loved one will kill themselves. Many of the caregivers I know are reluctant to address these issues, but in the end they have to face them.

Driving

Despite what we might believe, driving is a privilege and not a right. It is not about age; it is about being competent. A car is a two-thousand-pound weapon; it is no different from putting a loaded gun in someone's hand. I have seen clients who have difficulty picking up a pen or shuffling their feet in my office and who will (slowly and with great difficulty) make their way into the parking lot and get behind the wheel of a car. Some of the elderly have macular degeneration and can no longer see well. There are those who have some form of hearing impairment and can no longer hear a car horn, the squeal of brakes, or the sound of an approaching emergency vehicle. Every day the newspapers have stories about an accident that killed either the driver or other people. Some of the drivers were drinking, some were on medication, and some had dementia. Recently in New York, a man who had epilepsy and was on medication suffered a seizure while driving, lost control of his vehicle, and killed the three passengers in the car he hit.

As we age, some of us will naturally experience a slowing down of reaction time. If the person has any form of memory loss, driving can be deadly—not only for them but for innocent people. Many of my clients continue to allow the person with memory loss to drive for various reasons: they are afraid of the reaction the person might have if they are told not to drive, they do not want to take away the only independent activity the person still has, or they believe that if the person is told to stop driving, they will kill themselves. I have clients who say that they know that the person is having problems, so they limit their driving to familiar neighborhoods such as the grocery store, the golf course, or the hair salon. Their loved one should not be driving, but the caregiver continues to let them drive because it makes the caregiver's life easier.

There are people on the road today that should not be driving. When a person becomes confused in their home or wanders, they should not be behind the wheel of a car. The same goes for any person who has difficulty with new situations. Let's face facts: most of us drive on auto pilot. We use landmarks to guide us. "Go three blocks, and turn right at the pink house" is how many of us get around. What if the current owner decided to paint the pink house white? You or I might keep driving for a few more blocks and then realize that there was no pink house. A person with dementia will become so focused on the pink house they may not realize until miles, counties, or states later that they are no longer on course. If there is road construction or detours, a person with memory loss may find themselves in a dangerous neighborhood.

Some spouses tell me that their husband or wife still drives fine as long as they are with them in the car and give directions. The following is a true story as told to me by a daughter, who was in the car with her parents. Harry and Mary were going out for dinner as they had always done. The restaurant was local, just three miles away. Mary always directed Harry and told him where to stop, the color of the lights, and which way to turn. She would also guide him as to when it was safe to merge into another lane. This day while Harry was driving, Mary's purse opened up, and the contents spilled on the floor. She bent down to pick up her lipstick and took her eyes off the road. In a split second, Harry ran a red light, and their car was hit. Mary died.

For some, when they lack alternative reliable transportation, many people who have a form of memory loss will continue to drive. Often spouses continue to allow the person to drive because they themselves no longer feel comfortable behind the wheel. Maintaining independence is also a factor. My caregiver clients will ask me point blank when they should take away the car keys. There are several drawing tests that have shown to be a reliable indicator that the person is having visual and spatial problems. I have also found that your own gut feeling is a reliable tool—I call this the "family test." If the driver has difficulty staying in one lane and drifts into other lanes, drives too close to the curb, or has road rage, it is time to question their driving ability. If you feel any concern about the safety of letting your children, grandchildren, or great grandchildren in the car with this person, this is a perfect time to take away the car keys.

If you doubt the person's driving capabilities and need backup or reassurance, there are services that can evaluate their driving skills. I refer people to these services often. If the family is not open to my recommendation and insists that the person can continue to drive because they have no other way of getting around (or because taking away their independence "will kill them"), I tell them about the attorney rule: If the person has any form of dementia and gets into an accident, they and the family will and should be sued. This usually gets the family's attention.

Driving under the influence of alcohol or drugs is no different from operating a vehicle if you have a memory, vision, hearing, or gait impairment. This is not an elder issue; it's a safety issue. Medication may change your reaction time as well as cause fatigue, confusion, or dizziness. Some states now have a "duty to report" law that makes it mandatory for a doctor to report to the state when a person has dementia or memory loss. Check with your state to see if this law applies. Some doctors will report a person with dementia to their State Department Of Motor Vehicles even if their state does not have this law in order to protect the individual, the public, and themselves.

If despite knowing these factors you continue to let the person with dementia drive, to be on the safe side install a GPS tracking device in the car so that you can check where they have been, where they are going, and where their car is now. As the disorder progresses, there are things you can do to disable the car, such as flatten a tire, take out the spark plugs, or change the master key. If the car is parked in a garage, you can disable the garage door so that it appears to be broken and can't go up. I have advised clients to place the car "under repair" at the dealer. If the car is a lease, tell the person that the bank repossessed it because of lack of payment. You will need to take into consideration the level of dementia to make any of these tactics work.

Guns

A lot of people own guns. Many keep them in their homes or their car. They keep them for self-protection. Dementia and guns are a bad mix. The U.S. Constitution may allow for the right to bear arms, but there is nothing that addresses the situation when the person bearing arms is no longer competent. A gun in the hand of a person who has dementia is a safety issue. One of my clients did not recognize her husband, and mistaking him for an intruder, she shot him. Locate the guns, lock them up, and place the ammunition in a separate place. You can also sell them or give them away.

Wandering

This is one of the most misunderstood behavioral problems and one that happens most frequently. The person goes out to the driveway to pick up the mail or the newspaper, and once outside, they forget their purpose and just keep on going. If you are lucky, they will return home safely. Many people are not so lucky: they never find their way back home. With current technology, this doesn't need to happen. You can purchase small portable GPS devices and sew them or place them in the clothing of the person who has dementia that will track their whereabouts. If the person has a tendency to wander, or you are concerned that they may get lost, place the device in the clothes or purse that they are using today (just remember to remove it before you wash their clothes). You will now be able to track their location from your cell phone or by computer. Be aware that these devices are not foolproof.

There is a brand of sneaker on the market that has a built-in tracking device. It is designed to be used by a person who realizes they are lost and is capable of remembering to push the button on the shoe. A person in the moderate to severe stage of dementia most likely will not be able to remember to use this device if they get lost or are confused.

Before a person wanders, use common sense. Make sure that all doors and windows are secured. Keep on hand a current photo of the person. This will help when locating a missing person. Do not wait twenty-four hours to call the police; report a missing person who has dementia immediately. A person who wanders away will typically not answer to their name. They are scared and will find a hiding space that they feel is safe and hunker down. Just like a small child who is afraid of getting punished, the person with dementia will not respond to their name. Some will forget what their name is. Instead of saying Robert, use Bob or Bobby—a name the person might now recognize. A person with dementia may not realize the weather conditions and go out during a snow storm, hurricane or tornado. Anybody who has dementia should wear a Safe Return bracelet or necklace.

Eating

Do not allow a person with moderate to severe dementia to eat alone. They can put more food in their mouth than they are able to chew and swallow. Instead of spitting the food out, they will try to swallow and possibly choke in the process. This can be deadly. As this disorder progresses, many people lose the swallowing reflex and need to be constantly reminded. Keep the table simple, and only place out items that can be eaten. (One of my clients mistook the flower arrangement for a salad.) If a person is having swallowing problems, ask your doctor for a prescription for a speech/swallowing assessment.

Plants

Get rid of any plants that, although pretty, may be toxic. This is also a good time to remove any look-alike plants, shrubs, or bushes. In Florida, there are many plants that bloom with (inedible) fruit on them. At my summer home in Canada, there are many wild plants mixed in with blueberry and raspberry bushes that look similar but are poisonous. A person with dementia may see a blue plant on the ground and mistake it for blueberries.

Animals

Pets can be a great source of comfort to a person who has dementia; they give unconditional love and provide companionship. They can also keep the person active by requiring feeding and exercise. Animals give back to the person a sense of being responsible, a role that the elderly, because of their limited or reduced contact, often miss. A pet will also reduce social isolation. If you do not live with the person with dementia, be careful that the person does not over feed the pet. Remember that the person has memory loss and might forget that they just fed the pet. Dogs and fish will eat until their stomachs explode. Cats and birds will only eat when they are hungry. On the other extreme, a person with dementia may forget to feed their pets.

Know that cats may scratch, and a person who has dementia will have a compromised immune system. If a cat scratches you or me, we will easily recover; a person with dementia may become seriously ill. I am not a fan of cats being declawed, but there are many cats at animal shelters that have been declawed and are looking for a good home. To avoid respiratory infections, bird cages and cat litter boxes will need to be kept clean, and the dog should be regularly groomed.

Depending on where you live, fleas may be a problem. Where I live in South Florida, fleas are not seasonal—they are year-round. Flea bites can compromise the immune system of a person with dementia. Be smart, contract with an exterminator if a person has pets, or even if they don't, but they take daily walks outdoors. Fleas can jump on your clothing and be carried back into the home.

Socialization

People who are socially isolated decline quickly. Many of my clients who live alone have little human contact. They are not touched, spoken to, nor do they have any meaningful interactions with other people. They do not eat as well, exercise, or take their medication as prescribed, and they are not as mentally stimulated as those who live with another person, a family, or in an assisted living facility. The occasional or daily phone call or weekend visits are welcomed and enjoyed, but they do not address the solitary life of the elder.

If you care for your loved one from a distance, hiring a certified geriatric care manager will provide for socialization and manage your loved one's care while you are not with them. This will give you peace of mind, and allow you to live your life so that you are able to concentrate on your job and your family. The geriatric care manager will assess the current needs, give the family updates as to what is happening, and provide recommendations and suggestions to increase the person's quality of life. The fee is not covered by Medicare and is an out-of-pocket expense, although it may be tax deductible. An initial consultation depending on what is needed and where you live will cost from $100 to $250 per hour. An assessment of the home and living arrangements for a two hour visit with a complete report which includes recommendations will cost more. The fees for this type of service will range from $400 to $1,200, depending on where you live. This may sound like a lot of money but when you get back a good report for recommendations, referrals, activities, and follow up service- in the long run, this amount is nominal. You are getting an action care plan that you can use as a guide for the best care of your loved one. You get what you pay for.

As a geriatric social worker who specializes in dementia and a certified geriatric care manger, I go into the home for two hours, spend time with the caregivers and the family, assess the home and their environment which includes the family members and spend several hours writing up a solid care plan for the family based on their concerns, my observations, and recommendations. Once the family receives my care plan (which can also be sent to their family doctor or neurologist when requested), I take the time to review with the family their personal care plan. This follow up is included in my fee. For a person with dementia, a geriatric care manager may become a person that they can trust, have meaningful contact with, and introduce them to people and resources that they would not have had. For the family, the geriatric care manager will become a life line.

I can tell you that in order to keep the person that you care for functioning at a high level; you will need to engage your loved one in activities they will enjoy. As a caregiver you may say "no" to activities thinking that your loved one may not participate. The reality is that given a chance, the person that you care for will enjoy and benefit from attending a day center or local activities. The more a person interacts with others, the longer they will remain stable and have fewer behavioral problems. There are some people who I have met who refuse to leave their home or attend outside activities. Knowing in advance the level of dementia, I arrive at their home with a bag filled with appropriate activities. I open my bag and pull out items and start to engage with them. We play, laugh, and have fun. By the time I leave their home the family members and aides have a new direction and tools that they can use that will be emotionally and physically stimulating, engaging, inspiring, and increase socialization.

Long-Term Care Insurance

Once again, if you do not already have long-term care insurance, and you think that a person is having some form of memory loss, the most important thing that you can do is contact an insurance agent. Forget calling the neurologist's office and explaining that the person needs to see the doctor immediately; the person you need to contact before a diagnosis is a long-term care insurance agent. Once a person has a diagnosis of dementia, they will not be able to get coverage.

A person's age and any preexisting condition they have will affect the cost and coverage. The older the person is, the higher the monthly cost. Check with several companies, and then do the math. Each insurance company is different, and they will offer several different policies. Some companies will limit the total dollar amount that they will cover; other companies may have limited or unlimited benefits. Policies are often designed to provide and pay for specific care. Find out if the company will pay for a day center and an aide. Some will set a price for daily care. Anything over this amount will cost you out of pocket. Check to see what the hours a day is- some policies will charge per day as for services needed and others will charge off by the hour. Some policies are short term; others are for life. There are policies will pay for in home care, day centers, assisted living facility care and/or for care in a nursing home.

Speak with a financial advisor. Common sense says that even if a policy will cost you $10,000 dollars per year but the actual cost of care in your community is $100 dollars a day, this equals $36,000 dollars a year, and you are ahead of the game and saving $26,000 per year. If the actual cost of care is $250 dollars per day (which it is in many cities), your out-of-pocket expenses will be $80,000 per year. You have just saved $70,000 dollars. Unless a person is living in an assisted living facility or nursing home, these costs do not include their living arrangements. It is just for their care. If a person chooses to remain at home, you will need to factor in taxes, repairs, insurance, food, mortgage, and utility expenses.

No matter how great the policy looks or sounds, you need to do research on the insurance company. Long-term care insurance is just what it means: insurance for long-term care. Often these policies are bought years before they are needed or used. It is important to check the financial stability rating of the company and their current claim-paying history. Start your research with the *New York Times*. In 2007 and 2008 they did in-depth reports on long-term care policies. To be on the safe side, always check with the Better Business Bureau.

If you decide not to get insurance and feel that you can afford to pay for care yourself, be aware that the cost of caring for a person with dementia will depend on where they live and the type of care they will need. Plan on spending anywhere from $35,000 to $120,000 or more per year.

Medicare

When I meet with clients, I always ask them if they have long-term care insurance. Nine out of ten people will proudly say that they do because they have Medicare. Once again, you need to know that Medicare is health insurance, not long-term care insurance! Do not depend on Medicare to take of your loved one. Medicare will pay for hospital, medical, and rehabilitation expenses, up to a point. There are specific times and cost constraints for all of these services. Medicare is a federally administered health insurance program for a person who is sixty-five or older and is provided when Social Security benefits begin (unless a person has renal disease). Medicare will cover hospitalization (usually a hundred days) and certain services that the person may need to help them regain their previous functioning levels, such as physical, speech, and occupational therapies (for a limited time) as well as home health care and hospice care. With a prescription from a doctor, Medicare will pay for a hospital bed, wheelchair, and walker.

Medicare benefits are limited. Medicare has an 80/20 payout: it will pay 80 percent for care, and you are responsible for the cost of the additional 20 percent. As a consumer you need to know what your out-of-pocket costs will be. This is why HMOs are so popular. They claim to cover all of your health care needs from doctors to medication, as long as you stay within their plan. Read their contract carefully before signing on. When a person has dementia, an HMO may not be their best option. They will only be able to use the doctors currently within the plan (network), and it may be difficult to see any doctor or get a referral for a doctor or therapy that is outside the network. Some plans have limited benefits for specialists. The same goes for hospitals, rehabilitation, hospice, and some skilled nursing care facilities. Contact Medicare, and find out what it will pay for. No matter where you live, Medicare benefits will be the same because Medicare is universal in all states.

Here are the cliff notes for Medicare: It will be repetitive, since I covered this earlier in the book, but it is important for you to understand what is and isn't covered. Part A is hospitalization. Part B pays for doctor's visits and other types of outpatient care. Medigap is a supplemental insurance that is supposed to fill in the gaps of Medicare. Medigap has plans A through L and offers a different set of services, at a cost, depending on where you live. Medicare Part D is prescription coverage. Read the fine print; there are spending caps. There is a "doughnut hole," which is a gap that begins when your annual drug costs hit $2,700, and then you must pay all of the costs until you hit a certain limit. Once you hit the limit, prescription coverage will continue. If you purchase medications outside of the United States, it will not count for the doughnut hole. When it comes to drug plans, shop around. Compare what the plan charges for drugs that you are now using. Medicare Advantage plans, which are subsidized by the federal government and offered by insurance companies, are changing. Some plans are being eliminated, and the plan that you are on today may not be available during the next enrollment period. Check with Medicare to find out the current enrollment period.

Medicaid

If your loved one qualifies for Medicaid, let me just say, "Congratulations," because you have won the lottery. When you meet the financial qualifications for Medicaid, most of your medical care worries are now over. There are many government programs, institutional grants, and subsidies that will pay and provide for additional services that may be needed for their daily care. Medicaid will not provide for round-the-clock care, but it will provide for depending on need; aides for bathing, homemaker services, day center and meals. In addition, they can now go to any hospital, doctor, assisted living facility, or nursing home.

If the person qualifies for Medicaid, they may also be entitled to home-delivered meals or food stamps. Medicaid is the ultimate state-subsidized, long-term care plan. Medicaid is a federally aided, state-operated program that provides medical assistance to individuals and families who have limited resourccs. Unlike Medicare, where the benefits are the same in all fifty states, Medicaid benefits are different for each state. I have clients who have moved their loved one to another state because the qualifications and benefits were better.

For the moment, I want you to forget the word "Mcdicaid" and instead substitute the words "free aid." Many of my clients turn up their noses at Medicaid. They feel that there is a stigma attached to it because they have been taught that Medicaid is only for poor people. Wrong thinking! Medicaid is a government program that helps people who do not have thc ability to pay. What this means is that if you have limitcd assets and can qualify financially, the government will pick up your medical expenses with no premiums or deductibles. Medicaid will pick up the 20 percent of costs after Medicare, and if you qualify, it will pay 100 percent of your health care needs. Forget the stigma. Medicaid is thc only way to afford the cost of dementia care unless you are a millionaire or have good long-term care insurance.

With the help of a good financial planner and elder care attorney, you will be able to keep the assets that the person with dementia who has worked hard and long for and still qualify for Medicaid. I have clients who live at the most prestigious addresses and have Medicaid paying for aides for five or more hours (seven days a week), attending day centers, and all of their medical supplies, such as diapers, gloves, pads, and nutritional supplements. Timing and knowledge are everything when dealing with dementia. Had I had this knowledge years ago when my mother was first diagnosed, I may have been able to save some of her estate. Her private care cost over the last sixteen years has been astronomical. The reality is that the most expensive care for your loved one will come once they are in the middle to end stage of dementia. For many people, this can be the longest stage. With the right care, a person who is in the middle stage can live well for an additional eight to ten years or more. The more care needed, the higher the cost. To reduce these costs and protect your loved one's assets, hire a good elder care attorney.

In order to help you get over the stigma of Medicaid, let me tell you a story from a caregiver in one of the support groups I run. His mother had dementia and was placed in a nursing home. She had a roommate. They shared the same room and used the same aides, dining room, nurses, and doctor. They both received the same quality of care, but there was a difference: my friend paid out of pocket for his mother at a monthly cost of $6,000, and her roommate's family paid zero dollars because her care was covered by Medicaid. Caring for a person with dementia is expensive, especially if you don't have a good long-term care policy in place or good financial planning.

Financial Planning

Invest in a qualified competent elder care attorney. Years ago, nobody planned for dementia. My father had completed in writing all the financial planning that he felt would cover all of his family. The attorney agreed. Years later Dad died, and Mom had dementia. For the past seven years, she has been in the end stage of dementia. All of Dad's money has been spent on caring for Mom. I don't think that this was what he had planned. Until all of the money is used up, including her life insurance policy, which would have to be cashed out, she will not qualify for Medicaid. Since I am not an elder care attorney, I did not know this at the time. Obviously neither did our attorney—who came highly recommended—nor did our accountant, insurance agent, and financial consultant. No one knew that there were other financial care options. Years ago, nobody talked about dementia or estate planning for this disorder. Times have changed. Now that you know, you can make preparations for your financial future.

Trust me, what you spend now will save you money in the future. Hire a qualified elder care attorney who specializes in trusts and knows how best to qualify for Medicaid benefits in the present or, if needed, in the future. To financially and emotionally deal with dementia you will need a good financial plan that will save your money and ensure that your loved one receives government benefits even though it will cost you out of pocket today. Forget today, and think about tomorrow. Home care currently costs over $120 per day (this is on the low side). If you need two shifts of aides, it will cost you over $240 dollars per day. When it comes to paying for attorneys, do not be sticker-shocked by their fees. Many attorneys will charge a percentage of the estate, which is can range from three to five percent. Some attorneys may charge a flat fee.

Legal Documents

There are three documents everyone should have: a living will, a durable power of attorney, and a health care surrogate. All of these documents can be located online, but because states are different and have their own laws, it is best to have these documents prepared by a local elder care attorney (especially if you think they might be challenged). If your loved one lives out of state, check to make sure that these documents will be accepted and enforced in other states. A living will is a legal document that spells out what type of medical treatments you want and, most importantly, what you do not want to happen in the event that you are faced with a life-ending situation; if you have an incurable illness such as cancer or you are in a coma or have dementia. A living will carries out your personal wishes for future care when and if the need arises for procedures such as resuscitation (restarting the heart when it stops), feeding tubes (supplies nutrients through the stomach or nose), or other invasive or noninvasive medical procedures. A durable power of attorney is a document that gives another person the authority to act on your behalf and have the legal authority to pay your bills, transfer assets to pay for your care, sell or buy property, or donate to charities when you are no longer able to continue to do these things yourself. Basically, life will go on when you are not able. The third document that you should have is health care surrogate or medical power of attorney. This document allows a specified person to act on your behalf for your medical needs.

Know that if a person does not designate a health care surrogate the spouse is the first person recognized by the state to make medical decisions. After the spouse, children over 18 years old, then parents, siblings, cousins and lastly friends in this order is who will be designated by the courts as a viable surrogate. Even if a couple has been living together for years or they have a long term partnership (regardless of their sex), their relationship may not be recognized as valid. Every state has its own rules. No matter what your relationship is, to be safe, put in writing the person that you want as your health care surrogate. This will ensure that this person will be able to be there for you and ensure your health care decisions.

These three documents (living will, durable power of attorney and health care surrogate) will spell out your financial and medical wishes. You can find these documents online for a few dollars and download them, fill in the blanks, and sign them. For some people who have minimal or no assets, this might be the best route to go. I say "might" because each family is different and many of the forms are valid but generic, and may later cause a conflict over the estate. I recommend that you hire a qualified elder care attorney to draw up these documents to be sure that they will be valid.

As simple as these forms may seem, an elder care attorney will discuss each document at length with you. Remember, you are not only paying for the documents but also paying for their expertise. The $500 to $1,500 dollars you pay them may save you the $5,000 it would cost for you to go to court and file for guardianship in the future. A guardianship will restrain you from spending money on care unless it is approved by the courts. You will need to pay an attorney to represent you or the estate before you spend any money without the court's approval. I have a client with dementia who has been married for twenty-five years and has no children. He was paranoid and refused to sign the durable power of attorney. Over the past few years he has not done any repairs to the home (which is now falling down around him and his wife) and because of his memory disorder, he didn't want to spend the money and has missed payments on their homes (he has four) because they maintained separate checking accounts. Besides the $5,000 for the guardianship, she has spent over $15,000 in court fees just to present to the court the dire need for the home's repairs. To date, the judge has denied her requests. The judge has reduced every budget that my client has come up with. They used to travel four times a year, and their judge will not budget for this. (Not all judges are unreasonable; however, once your case is in the legal system, you never know what judge is going to have power over your and your loved one's lives.) Through coaching, my client's wife has become stronger. She doesn't want to leave her husband, but if she does, the estate will have to pay for a full-time caregiver. This is not what her husband would have ever wanted. Had he known, he might have signed the durable power of attorney if it was explained in a way and by a person that made him comfortable.

Be very careful when it comes to filling out and signing a durable power of attorney form. There is now a limited durable power form that does just what the name says: it limits what another person (usually the children) can do with the assets depending on the cognitive or physical impairment of the assignee.

Ask your attorney about a limited power of attorney. This may never happen to you, but the following happened to a couple as told to me by one of my attorney friends. Bill and Mary (both cognitively normal) went to their family attorney to do estate planning, and on the advice of their attorney, they gave their oldest married son, Mark (the father of their only grandchild), durable power of attorney. When they came back from their holiday and opened the mail, they discovered that two of their brokerage accounts had been closed and the money removed. Turns out that Mark's wife convinced him that they deserved the money and encouraged Mark to remove the funds from the account. Needless to say, Bill and Mary had no legal recourse. Once they signed the durable power of attorney form, Mark had legal access to all of their funds. Bill and Mary found an estate attorney and changed their power of attorney to a different child. Needless to say, they not only were devastated by the financial loss but suffered an emotional loss as well. They no longer communicate with this son or their grandchild.

The vast majority of caregivers will not take advantage of their position or the trust of their loved one. You should also keep in mind that over time, laws will change. You should review and update the documents every three to five years. You may want to change some of the people you once named on the documents; perhaps they are no longer available or able to carry out your wishes. You should also include the names of one or two doctors who need to state your competence before the document can be enforced. Keep all of your forms handy so that you can bring them to the emergency room or hospital. Once again, a limited power of attorney will do just that, limit access to specific accounts. A durable power of attorney gives unlimited access to everything.

The reality is that care costs, and good care costs more. The price of in-home care for a person with dementia is expensive. As the disease progresses, the cost will rise. Facilities factor in these costs, and if you are caring for a person in your home, you need to do the same. Facility costs will charge for taxes and insurance rates as well as costs of building maintenance and personal care. Factor in repairs to your home if the person with dementia is now living there. When I first bought my home eight years ago, the windstorm insurance was $1,900. Last year the windstorm insurance bill cost over $8,000. Over the past sixteen years the cost of caring for Mom has risen dramatically. The taxes I pay because of the housing boom have tripled. My salary has not. Be smart· Take into account a cost of living increase and an increase in insurance (life, long-term care, homeowners, flood, car, windstorm, etc.) in your financial plan, as well as the costs of caring for your loved one. Tax laws change yearly. You should add to your team a knowledgeable accountant to help you.

Hospice Care

Hospice is the least used and most misunderstood form of end-of-life care, especially when it comes to a person who has dementia. People often think that hospice is only for those who have six months or less to live. This is not always the case when it comes to dementia. Hospice care is paid out of Medicare or Medicaid. Hospice will provide doctors, nurses, social workers, and aides; physical, speech, or occupational therapy; pet therapy, massage, musical therapy, and medication, as well as diapers, gloves, bed liners, beds, and air mattresses. Hospice will provide for everything that is medically, emotionally, and physically needed. It can send a chaplain or rabbi to the person's home for their spiritual needs. Talk about one-stop shopping!

Many people are turned off by hospice because they believe that once hospice comes in, the person they love is going to die. Nothing can be further from the truth. The services that hospice provides can actually increase the quality of life for the person who has dementia and that of the family. I know many clients who have improved with the care they received from hospice. Hospice is not a place; it is a service. Hospice care is provided in your home or wherever the person is living now. If your loved one is in an assisted living facility or nursing home, hospice will go there too.

Hospice provides all of the medical care your loved one requires. When a person qualifies for hospice, there is nothing more that your neurologist or doctor can do. The best care will be given by the hospice team. I can tell you this because my mother, while in the severe end stage of dementia, was placed over four years ago on hospice and was discharged on two different occasions. According to hospice, she "wasn't declining" fast enough. Mom went through two different hospices, and even in her severe state, she had a slow decline—but still hung on. When the time comes, the care that hospice will provide will add to the quality of life for the person who is being cared for and the family.

Brain Donation

The organ donor foundations have done a wonderful job of educating the public about the benefits of organ donation. Every year, many lives are lost through tragic events. Organ donations are a gift that allows many people the chance of a normal life. Until I worked at my center, I had never heard about brain donation. I knew about eyes, hearts, kidneys, and skin, to name just a few of the organs that can be donated to help another person live a better life, but brain donation was new to me. Brain donation is a twofold gift. For the family who has dealt with dementia for so long, they now will have a definite diagnosis. I hear from some people, "The doctor said she had Alzheimer's disease, so why should I bother?" Doctors can be wrong and misdiagnose dementia. It is not unusual for a family to believe that their loved one had Alzheimer's, but after the autopsy it turns out that they had a different type of dementia. Remember, there are eighty-six different types of dementia, and Alzheimer's is just one of them. Some types may be reversed or avoided through lifestyle and environmental changes. An autopsy can help future generations of the family to plan for their own long-term care. For researchers, brain donation will help them better understand dementia, which may lead to a cure. Brain donation is a win-win situation.

Taking Time Off

If you are still working, you should go to your company's Human Resource (HR) department and find out if they comply with the Family Medical Leave Act (FMLA). Companies with over fifty employees are legally obligated to follow FMLA. FMLA entitles you to three months of leave to care for yourself or a family member. Get the forms, fill them out, and send them to the neurologist or primary doctor to fill out and sign, and then have them faxed or mailed back to your HR department. This form is legal protection that will allow you time off from work without the threat of being fired while you care for your loved one.

Many workplaces have a fire-at-will policy. If you need to take time off for a period of time, like caring for a family member, you could be dismissed from your job. FMLA can protect you. Even if your coworkers are understanding and you work for the best boss in the world, you could be at risk, and this document will give you a legal edge. Depending on the company, your time-off pay may come out of your vacation or paid time-off days that you have accumulated. Once you have exceeded this time, you will no longer be paid, but you will still have your benefits (like insurance). Some companies will hold your job for you until you return; other employers may assign you to a different department.

You do not have to take three months off all at once to benefit from FMLA. It will also allow you to take intermittent time off to attend to doctor's appointments or provide assistance. Typically I help only a handful of caregiver clients fill out these forms each year. During my intake interview with clients I address family leave. Many of my clients have never heard of it or mistakenly believe that it is just for pregnant women or parents of newborn babies. Caring for a person with dementia is included in FMLA. If your company provides for family leave, you are entitled and should use this benefit.

CHAPTER TWELVE

A FINAL THOUGHT ABOUT CAREGIVING

I always believed that my parents alone raised me. Having an opportunity to look back and review, I now know that my parents used the guidance of their village to help them.

In the 1930s, my father, an avid outdoorsman and hunter, ended up in a remote village in Canada: Sheahan, Ontario. With his best friend Jack, a Canadian furrier, the two of them set out into the wilderness to go for big game—bear and moose. Despite being successful in their professions and good hunters in Pennsylvania and Ontario (and fortunately for the wildlife in Canada), they came home with nothing.

Dad realized that he couldn't do it on his own. He would need a guide to help him. After asking the locals for advice, Dad hired Otto, a Canadian Indian, who guided him in the woods and taught my father how to successfully hunt in this unfamiliar land. With Otto as his guide, my father got the game he wanted. Through their adventures, Otto became my father's friend and trusted guide in the Canadian outback. Based on Otto's advice, my father bought land on Lake Pogamasing, where they built a log cabin as a base camp for their fall and spring hunting trips. Years later, Otto and my father built the main lodge from trees on the property.

This became the camp where I spent my childhood summers. Growing up, I spent three months of the year far removed from civilization. There were no cars or roads, phones, electricity, indoor plumbing, or running water. The nearest family is miles away by boat. The only access is by train or seaplane. To get to the train it means going miles by boat on open waters to get to the landing, walking almost a mile through the woods, taking a boat across the river, and walking a quarter of a mile to the train tracks. We have a train that's called the "Bud Car," which, when not on strike, runs between Sudbury and Timmons. I remember summers when the train ran daily between towns. Because of budget cuts, the rail service changed, and the train ran (and still runs) every other day—except on Monday, when there is no rail service. In an emergency, you need to stand on the train track and use a flashlight to stop a freight train to take you into town. Picture yourself sitting in a one-room train station shack, listening for the sound and feeling the changing movement of the ground to know when a train is coming. I know what it is like to be in the wilderness, in total darkness, waiting to flag down a freight train. Isolation breeds dependency on others. From a very young age I was taught the importance of survival, teamwork, and having a really good guide.

My father taught me wilderness survival skills, as did the Indians from the nearest lodges and the locals who lived on the lake year-round or seasonally. I learned from the tribal elders how to locate and fall the trees that I would need to repair the camp or build a dock or water tower. I was taught how to recognize berries that I could eat and which to avoid, and most importantly how to safely find my way back home should I get lost (which I did quite a few times). I learned the importance of working with what you have and reaching out to others when needed. To eat, you need to fish. In order to fish, you need to know where the fish are. No matter how good a fisherman you are in your own back yard, each area of the lake is different and you will need the help of a guide to show you the best place to catch fish. These are not everyday skills that a girl from Miami Beach will need to survive in the city, but they were tools to help me survive in the woods.

The lake is about forty miles long with wide bays, narrows, channels, shoals and big rocks. There are thirty cottages on the lake (some clustered together, others miles apart) and some families, like mine, have been here for more than seventy years. Everyone looks out for everyone else. The landscape of the lake is constantly changing due to nature and the dam. Neither, can we control. Some summers we have a beach, and other times the water comes up to or over the shore line. As camp people, we learn to adapt. Some of us build on to our docks, others build new trails to dock the boats, and some will tie their boat to the nearest tree and walk through the water. When we get together as a village, we will gripe and complain about the situation, and band together against the dam ("Damn the dam"), even though for some of us the water level is now in our favor.

The lessons the elders on the lake instilled in me are the lessons that have been the guiding force in my life: share your knowledge, ask others for help, and learn by watching others and letting others watch you. It doesn't matter whether you live in a big city or in the Canadian outback; in order to get through difficult moments, you will need the guidance and the wisdom of a village.

Compared to survival in the outback, dementia is the tougher situation to deal with. Mom passed away on July 26, 2009—Dad's birthday. When Mom passed, this book was being edited. When I got it back for approval, there were sections I decided not to change. My mother has been with me for many years, and even with her passing, she is still with me. I keep the light on in her bedroom, which gives me comfort when I spend time outside or look out my bedroom window at night. I know that she is no longer here, but for a few moments, seeing her light allows me to believe that she is still home with me. The loss from her passing continues. Caring for Mom was a big part of my life. My life and my children's lives revolved around her and her care, and now that she is gone, there is a huge void. For me, the sacrifices I made were worthwhile: despite what I went through caring for Mom, I would do it again. If I had better guidance—like what is in this book—my life, her life, and my family's life would have been better and easier.

Since Mom's death, I have had a chance to reflect on the lessons I learned through the past twenty-five years of caring for her. There were times when caring for my mother was a daily challenge. There were times when I needed to flag down a freight train. For our survival, I pulled from all of the resources that were available to me. In times of crisis, I did the best with what I had and received guidance from those who were experts in their field. I did not care for my mother alone; I reached out to the village to help me. No matter where we live, we have a village; family, friends, professionals and the internet can help us. As caregivers we need to reach out and ask for help.

RESOURCES

Alzheimer's Disease Research Centers

Below is a list of Alzheimer's disease research centers organized by state. They are a good source to contact about memory disorder clinics in your state and have valuable information about clinical trials and other resources. This information was accurate at the time this book was published.

ALABAMA
Alzheimer's Disease Research Center
University of Alabama
Sparks Research Center
1720 7th Avenue South, Suite 650K
Birmingham, AL 35233-7340
www.uab.edu/adc
205-934-3847
e-mail: dmarson@uab.edu

ARIZONA
Arizona Alzheimer's Disease Center/
Sun Health Research Institute
Banner Alzheimer's Institute
901 East Willeta Street
Phoenix, AZ 85006
www.azalz.org
602-239-6525

ARKANSAS
University of Arkansas for Medical Sciences
Alzheimer's Disease Center
Donald W. Reynolds Department of Geriatrics
4301 West Markham, Slot 808
Little Rock, AR 72205-7199
http://alzheimer.uams.edu
501-603-1294

CALIFORNIA
Stanford University
Stanford/ VA Alzheimer's Disease Center
Department of Psychiatry, 5550
401 Quarry Road, C305
Stanford, CA 94305-5717
http://alzheimer.stanford.edu
650-852-3287
e-mail: amott@stanford.edu

University of California, Davis
Alzheimer's Disease Center
4860 Y Street, Suite 3700
Sacramento, CA 95817-4540
http://alzheimer.ucdavis.edu
916-734-5496

University of California, Irvine
Alzheimer's Disease Research Center
Gillespie Neuroscience Research Facility, Room 1113
Irvine, CA 92697-4540
www.alz.uci.edu
949-824-5847

University of California, Los Angeles
Alzheimer's Disease Center
10911 Weyburn Avenue, Suite 200
Los Angeles, CA 90095-1769
www.adc.ucla.edu
Information on research studies
and clinical trials: 310-206-6397

University of California, San Diego
Alzheimer's Disease Research Center
Department of Neurosciences
UCSD School of Medicine
9500 Gilman Drive (0624)
La Jolla, CA 92093-0624
http://adrc.ucsd.edu
858-622-5800
e-mail: adrc@ucsd.edu

University of California, San Francisco
Alzheimer's Disease Research Center
350 Parnassus Avenue, Suite 706
San Francisco, CA 94143-1207
http://memory.ucsf.edu
415-476-6880
e-mail: adrc@memory.ucsf.edu

University of Southern California
Alzheimer's Disease Research Center
Health Consultation Center
1510 San Pablo Street, HCC643
Los Angeles, CA 90033
www.usc.edu/dept/gero/ADRC
213-740-7777
e-mail: uscadrc@usc.edu

FLORIDA
Florida Alzheimer's Disease Research Center/ Byrd Alzheimer's Institute
15310 Amberly Drive, Suite 320
Tampa, Fl 33647
www.floridaadrc.org
866-700-7773
Director's e-mail: hpotter@byrdinstitute.org

GEORGIA
Emory University
Alzheimer's Disease Center
Neurology Department
101 Woodruff Circle, #6000
Atlanta, GA 30322
www.med.emory.edu/ADC
404-728-6950

ILLINOIS
Northwestern University
Cognitive Neurology and Alzheimer's Disease Center
Feinberg School of Medicine
675 North St. Claire, Galter 20-100
Chicago, IL 60611
www.brain.northwestern.edu
312-908-9339
e-mail: CNADC-Admin@northwestern.edu
Director's e-mail: mmesulam@northwestern.edu

Rush University Medical Center
Alzheimer's Disease Center
Armour Academic Center

600 South Paulina Street, Suite 1028
Chicago, Il 60612
312-942-2362

INDIANA
Indiana University School of Medicine
Indiana Alzheimer Disease Center
Department of Pathology and Lab Medicine
635 Barnhill, Drive, MS-A-138
Indianapolis, IN 46202-5120
http://iadc.iupui.edu
317-278-5500
e-mail: iadc@iupui.edu

KENTUCKY
University of Kentucky
Alzheimer's Disease Center
Sanders- Brown Center on Aging, Room 101
800 South Limestone Street
Lexington, KY 40536-0230
www.mc.uky.edu/coa
859-323-6040

MARYLAND
John Hopkins University
Alzheimer's Disease Research Center
Division of Neuropathology
558 Ross Research Building
720 Rutland Avenue
Baltimore, MD 21205-2196
www.alzresearch.org
410-502-5164

MASSACHUSETTS
Boston University
Alzheimer's Disease Center
Bedford VA Medical Center
GRECC Program (182B)
200 Springs Road
Bedford, MA 01730
www.bu.edu/alzresearch
617-638-5368
e-mail: decart@bu.edu

**Massachusetts General Hospital /
Harvard Medical School**
Alzheimer's Disease Research Center
114 16th Street, Room 2009
Charlestown, MA 02129
http://madrc.org
617-726-3987

MICHIGAN
University of Michigan
Alzheimer's Disease Research Center
Department of Neurology
300 North Ingalls, Room 3D15
Ann Arbor, MI 48109-0489
www.med.umich.edu/alzheimers
734-764-2190
e-mail: neuro-ADresearch@med.umich.edu

MINNESOTA
Mayo Clinic
Alzheimer's Disease Research Center
Department of Neurology

200 First Street, SW
Rochester, MN 55905
http://mayoresearch.mayo.edu/mayo/
research/alzheimers_center
507-284-1324
e-mail: mayoADC@mayo.edu

MISSOURI
Washington University School of Medicine
Alzheimer's Disease Research Center
Department of Neurology
4488 Forest Park Avenue, Suite 130
St. Louis, MO 63108-2293
http://alzheimer.wustl.edu
Research participation and questions: 314-286-2683
Education and rural outreach: 314-286-2882
 or 286-0930

NEW YORK
Columbia University
Alzheimer's Disease Center
630 West 168 Street, P&S 15-402
New York, NY 10032
www.alzheimercenter.org
212-305-1818

Mount Sinai School of Medicine
Alzheimer's Disease Research Center
Department of Psychiatry
One Gustave Levy Place, Box 1230
New York, NY 10029-6574
www.mssm.edu/psychiatry/adrc
212-241-8329

New York University
Alzheimer's Disease Center
ADRC, Millhauser Labs
560 First, Avenue
New York, NY 10016
www.med.nyu.edu/adc
212-263-8088

NORTH CAROLINA
Duke University Medical Center
Joseph and Kathleen Bryan
Alzheimer's Disease Research Center
2200 West Main Street, Suite A-230
Durham, NC 27705
http://adrc.mc.duke.edu
866-444-2372 (toll free)

OREGON
Oregon Health and Science University
Aging and Alzheimer's Disease Center CR 131
3181 SW Sam Jackson Park Road
Portland, OR 97239-3098
www.ohsu.edu/research/alzheimers
503-494-6976

PENNSYLVANIA
University of Pennsylvania School of Medicine
Alzheimer's Disease Center
Department of Pathology and Laboratory Medicine
HUP, Maloney 3rd Floor
36th and Spruce Streets
Philadelphia, PA 19104-4283
www.uphs.upenn.edu/ADC
215-662-7810

University of Pittsburgh
Alzheimer's Disease Research Center
Department of Neurology
3471 Fifth Avenue, Suite 811
Pittsburgh, PA 15213- 2582
www.adrc.pitt.edu
412-692-2700

TEXAS
University of Texas, Southwestern Medical Center
Alzheimer's Disease Research Center
Department of Neurology
5323 Harry Lines Boulevard
Dallas, TX 75390-9036
www.utsouthwestern.edu/alzheimers/research
214-648-9376

WASHINGTON
University of Washington
Alzheimer's Disease Center
VA Puget Sound Health Care System
Mental Health Services, S-116
1660 South Colombian Way
Seattle, WA 98108
www.depts.washington.edu/edrcweb
206-277-3281

Phones for People with Dementia

For any of the phones listed below, search on
the name in an online search engine (e.g.,
search "GE PhotoPhone" in Google).

In-Home Phones

General Electric (GE) makes PhotoPhone, which
has a caller ID that shows not only who is calling
but also a photo ID. It's an all-in-one landline.

Radio Shack makes a picture phone that can do one-
touch calling based on the picture of the person.

The Alzheimer's Store has a host of products and
solutions for people with dementia and their caregivers.
Go to www.alzstore.com or call 1-800-752-3238.

Cell Phones with Tracking Devices

The Disney Family Locator service on the Disney-
branded mobile phone uses a GPS (global positioning
system) to track a person's whereabouts.

Sprint has a family locator service that provides
a person's location and alerts the family member
when the person arrives at a specified place.

Verizon's child locator, called Chaperone,
has a perimeter program, and an alert is sent
if a person leaves the defined area.

Wherify Wireless has a GPS-enabled phone
that makes tracking a person easy.

People Track USA: Call 1-866-618-
9238 or www.trackmykids.com.

Easy-to-Use Cell Phones

Samsung Jitterbug phone: www.jitterbugphone.
com or call 1-800-918-8543.

Verizon's Wireless Coupe: www.verizon.com.

Other Devices that Keep the Elder Safe from Afar

Brickhouse Security (www.brickhousesecurity.
com): One-stop shopping for GPS devices.
They have a live-wire lightning device that keeps
a ninety-day record of all vehicle travel.

Pocket Finders (globalsources.com) is a GPS
device that lets you locate the holder anywhere
by way of the internet. You can also designate
safety zones, and if a person is driving, it will
track how fast the person is driving.

Project Lifesaver (www.projectlifesaver.com;
1-877-580-5433). Their device can locate your
loved one within moments if they wander away.

Safety Net by LoJack (www.lojacksafetynet.com or
call 1-877-434-6384). They have an electronic search
and rescue bracelet that is worn on wrist or ankle.

Resources for Caregiving Contracts, Financial Planning, and Related Issues

American Bar Association Commission on Law and Aging: www.abanet.org/aging

Family Caregiver Alliance: www.caregiver.org

Financial Planning Association: 1-800-282-7526 or 1-800-322-4237.
National Academy of Elder Law Attorneys: www.Naela.com

National Family Caregivers Association: www.thefamilycaregiver.org

Advocates and Ombudsman Programs

American Association of Retired Persons (AARP): www.aarp.org

Assisted Living Federation of America: www.alfa.org

Consumer Consortium on Assisted Living: www.ccal.org

The Eldercare Locator: This links caregivers with senior services and other community resources. 1-800-677-1116 or www.aoa.dhhs.gov or www.eldercare.gov.

National Association for Assisted Living: www.ncal.org

National Association of Geriatric Care Managers: Geriatric care managers can help make your life easier, from assessing the elder's current and long-term care needs, to assisting with placement in a care facility and helping you navigate the health care system. This will give you peace of mind and save you time and money. 520-881-8008 or www.caremanager.org.

National Association of Social Workers: www.nasw.com.

National Association of Units on Aging: Each state has an office of the long-term care ombudsman program. 202-898-2578 or www.ltombudsman.org.

Background Checks

Intelius: www.intelius.com

Personal Remote Emergency Response System

These system offers a quick response for loved ones who live alone or may be left alone for periods of time. Some may be able to place motion detectors in the home:

ADT Home Health Security Services: 1-877-238-3880 or www.ADT.com.

Alert Sentry: 1-877-253-7899 or www.alertsentry.com.

Lifefone: 1-800-331-9198 or www.lifefone.com.

Philips Lifeline: 1-800-451-0525 or www.lifelinesystems.com.

The Cast Clearinghouse: www.agingtech.org

The Quiet Care system: 1-866-216-4600 or www.quietcaresystems.com

Government Programs and Health Insurance

Eldercare Locator: This service of the U.S. Administration on Aging is funded by the federal government and provides information and referrals to respite care and other home and community services. 1-800-677-1116 or www.eldercare.gov Also check out their Prescription Drug Options for Older Adults.

Foundation for Health Coverage Education: Twenty-four-hour helpline 1-800-234-1317 or www.coverageforall.org.

Genworth Financial (longtermcare.genworth.com) has a 2007 cost-of-care survey on their website.

Medicare and Medicaid: www.medicare.gov.

National Institute of Health: www.nihseniorhealth.gov.

Medication Management

American Medical Alert (www.age-in-place.com) has Med-Time.

Timex (www.timexhealthcare.com) has a daily medication manager.

Lost Item Location Devices

Loc8tor (www.loc8tor.com) can find up to seven items that are misplaced up to six hundred feet away. The cost starts at $100.

Sharper Image (www.sharperimage.com) has a great remote key locator.

Light Therapy

The following resources can help someone cope with Seasonal Affective Disorder, sundown syndrome, or sleep problems.

The Center for Environmental Therapies (www.cet.org) sells light boxes for $200.

Philips Go Lite Blu: www.lighttherapy.com

Sunrise Systems Lightbox: www.sadlight.com

Government Agencies and Nonprofit Organizations

The Administration on Aging (AOA): A one-stop service that links seniors to services in the community. 202-619-0724 or www.aoa.gov.

Aging with Dignity: They publish the Five Wishes Living Will document, which meets the legal requirements in thirty-five states. 888-594-7437 or www.agingwithdignity.org.
 The Alzheimer's Association: They support families and caregivers of people with Alzheimer's disease and have chapters nationwide that provide referrals to local resources. They also sponsor support groups and educational programs. Twenty-four-hour hotline 1-800-272-3900 or www.alz.org.

Alzheimer's Disease Education and Referral Center (ADRC): Very informative and good start for research studies. They have publications on diagnosis, treatment, medication, patient care, caregiver needs, and long-term care. 1-800-438-4380 or www.cais.net/adear or www.nia.nih.gov.

American Association of Homes and Services for the Aging: Free information on long-term care and housing. 202-783-2242 or www.aahsa.org.

American Association of Retired Persons (AARP): A leading organization for people age fifty and older and a one-stop information source., including information on health insurance and medication. 1-800-424-3410 or www.aarp.com.

American Medical Association: They provide physician referrals and have good information on medications. 1-312-464-5000 or www.ama-aasn.org.

The Association for Frontal Temporal Dementias: www.aftd.org or www.ftd-picks.org.

Department of Veterans Affairs (VA): If your loved one was in the military, you need to check out this site. They are slow in processing claims or getting disability, and you will need to be persistent. 1-800-827-1000 or 1-877-222-8387 or www.va.gov.

Family Caregiver Alliance: They offer programs at the national, state, and local levels to support caregivers. 1-415-434-3388 or www.caregiver.org.

National Alliance for Caregiving (NAC): This group supports caregivers and teaches about issues facing caregivers today. 1-301-718-8444 or www.caregiving.org.

National Association for Home Care: They have material to help you select a home health care agency. 1- 202-547-7424 or www.nahc.org.

National Council on Aging (NCOA): They have information about respite care. Their "Benefits Check Up" website helps you find government and private programs that serve seniors. 1-800-375-1014 or www.ncoa.org or benefitscheckup.org.

National Hospice and Palliative Care Organizations: They offer information on end-of-life issues and state-specific advance directives. 1-800-658-8898 or www.nhpco.org.

National Institute on Aging: They have free publications available in both English and Spanish on different topics of aging. Call 1-800-222-2225 or go to www.nia.nih.gov

National Parkinson's Foundation: They provide information and medical support. 1-800-327-4545 or www.parkinson.org.
National Stroke Association: They provide information and referrals to local stroke support groups. 1-800-787-6537 or www.stroke.org.

Nursing Home Compare: They provide detailed information on the past performance of every Medicare- and Medicaid-certified nursing home in the United States. www.medicare.gov/nhcompare.

Social Security: There may be a larger monthly benefit for applying for its Supplemental Security Income (SSI) program. It's worth checking out. www.socialsecurity.gov.

United States Administration on Aging: The official federal agency dedicated to the delivery of supportive and community-based services. Check out the website's section on family caregiving. 202-619-0724 or www.aoa.gov or www.govbenefits.gov.

United States Department of Justice: Learn about
disabilities (and dementia is one). This website offers
information and free publications on the regulations
to grant universal access to people with disabilities.
www.ada.gov/publicat.htm#anchor-14210.

Drug Assistance Programs and Information

AARP has an online calculator that will let you know
how much you will have to pay out of pocket before you
hit the "donut hole". Go to www.aarp.org/doughnuthole

Access to Benefits: Search for public and private
programs. www.accesstobenefits.org.

Administration on Aging: Drug assistance programs
run by states. 1-800-677-1116 or www.eldercare.gov.

Benefits Check Up RX: This site provides a free
personal report, once you fill out a questionnaire that
will tell you all of the prescription drug programs
you are eligible for. www.benefitscheckuprx.com.

Best Pills Worst Pills is a good resource for an
independent first or second opinion when it comes to
prescription drug information. www.worstpills.org.

Consumer Reports: Learn more about saving money
on prescription drugs. www.crbestbuydrugs.org.

Drug guide that lists side effects and links to
support groups. www.Drugs.com/sfx

Food and Drug Administration: Current FDA medication safety information: www.fda.gov/prescriptionhelp/. Learn about buying drugs online: www.fda.gov/buyonline. For assistance from pharmaceutical companies.

The National Association of Boards of Pharmacy reviews websites that sell medications and lists accredited sites. www.nabp.net.

NeedyMeds.com: Find out about state programs, discount drug cards, federal guidelines, and assistance programs. www.needymeds.com. Partnership for Prescription Assistance: This site includes more than 475 public and private pharmaceutical programs. You can search for programs and also get assistance with Medicare Part D. 1-888-477-2669 or www.pparx.org.

Pharmaceutical Research and Manufacturers of America: They have a website that lists patient assistance programs. www.helpingpatients.org.

Pharmacy Checker: Check out and compare prescription drug prices for more than one thousand medications. www.PharmacyChecker.com

Rate A Drug: prescription drugs and alternative treatments. www.RateADrug.com View or submit ratings on effectiveness and side effects of over 8,000.

Rx Assist: Find drug assistance programs. www.rxassist.com.

Side effects of popular drugs: They have a list of
most drugs that are commonly prescribed and
explain the purpose of the drug. www.RxList.com

Social Security Administration: Online
help with prescription drug costs. www.
socialsecurity.gov/prescriptionhelp.

Together Rx: A good source for prescription
drugs if you do not have insurance. 1-800-
444-4106 or www.togetherrxaccess.com.
Web MD: An easy to use data base of drugs, effectiveness
and their side effects. Go to www.Webmd.com

Some additional portals that you might want to check
out are: www.rxhope.com, www.needymeds.org, www.
patientassistance.com, www.patientadvocate.org, and the
Partnership for Prescription Assistance (www.pparx.org).

Dietary Supplements

Before you use or continue to use any dietary
supplements you should speak with your doctor.
Below are some websites that may be useful:

National Library of Medicine's Medline Plus.
Go to medlineplus.gov, under Drugs and
Supplements: http/www.nim.nih.gov

National Center for Complimentary and
Alternative Medicine: http://nccam.nih.gov

Office of Dietary Supplements: http://
dietary-supplements.info.nih.com

The Centers for Disease Control and Prevention: http://
www.cdc.gov/nutrition/everyone/basics/vitamins.

Caregiving Contracts

These sites have information on caregiving
contracts and caregiving issues:

National Academy of Elder Law
Attorneys: www.naela.com

American Bar Association Commission on
Law and Aging: www.abanet.org/aging

National Family Caregivers Association:
www.thefamilycaregiver.org

Family Caregiver Alliance: www.caregiver.org

National Alliance for Caregiving: www.caregiving.org

Online Wills

Build A Will: www.buildawill.com

Legacy Writer: www.Legacywriter.
com or call 888-609-3474

Legal Zoom: www.legalzoom.com

Susie Orman's Will and Trust kit: www. suzeormanwillandtrust.com

Organizational Tools

These systems offer computer software to assist the caregiver in organizing, storing and sharing important documents and information:

Caregiver's Touch: www.cargiverstouch.com

Care Binders: www.carebinders.com or call 201-447-1577

Recommended Reading

Beckerman, Anita G., and Ruth M. Tappen. *It Takes More Than Love: A Practical Guide to Taking Care of an Aging Adult*. Baltimore: Health Professions Press, 2000.

Beckwith, Bill E. *Managing Your Memory: Practical Solutions for Forgetting*. Fort Myers, FL: Memory Management, 2004.

Castleman, Michael, Dolores Gallagher-Thompson, and Matthew Naythons. *There's Still a Person in There: The Complete Guide to Treating and Coping with Alzheimer's*. New York: Putnam, 1999.

Feil, Naomi. *V/F Validation: The Feil Method: How to Help Disoriented Old-Old*. Rev. ed. Cleveland: Edward Feil Productions, 1992.

Gillick, Muriel R. *Tangled Minds: Understanding Alzheimer's Disease and Other Dementias.* New York: Dutton, 1998.

Mendez, Mario F., and Jeffrey L. Cummings. *Dementia: A Clinical Approach.* 3rd ed. Philadelphia: Butterworth-Heinemann, 2003.

Radin, Lisa. *What If It's Not Alzheimer's? A Caregiver's Guide to Dementia.* New York: Prometeus, 2003.

Small, Gary. *The Memory Bible: An Innovative Strategy for Keeping Your Brain Young.* New York: Hyperion, 2002.

Strauss, Claudia J. *Talking to Alzheimer's: Simple Ways to Connect When You Visit with a Family Member or Friend.* Oakland, CA: New Harbinger Publishers, 2001.

Today's Caregiver. Founded by Gary Barg, this magazine is filled with helpful information covering a range of topics as well as information about the Fearless Caregiver Conference. Call 1-800-829-2734 or 954-893-0550, or go to www.caregiver.com.

United Kingdom and International Resources

Alzheimer's Disease International (ADI) is the international federation of 71 national Alzheimer's Associations around the world: www.alz.co.uk

Alzheimer Society is the leading UK organization and will provide information, support and referrals to appropriate organizations: call the helpline at 0845-300-0336 or +44(0)-20-7423-3500 or go to their website www.alzheimersorg.uk

INDEX